SECOND LIVES,
SECOND CHANCES

SECOND LIVES,
SECOND CHANCES

*A Surgeon's Stories
of Transformation*

Donald R. Laub, MD

Published by ECW Press
665 Gerrard Street East
Toronto, ON M4M 1Y2
416-694-3348 / info@ecwpress.com

Cover design: David A. Gee
Cover photo: From the author's personal
collection

PRINTED AND BOUND IN CANADA

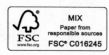

To the best of his abilities, the author has related
experiences, places, people, and organizations
from his memories of them. In order to protect
the privacy of others, he has, in some instances,
changed the names of certain people and details
of events and places.

LIBRARY AND ARCHIVES CANADA CATALOGUING
IN PUBLICATION

Laub, Donald R., author
    Second lives, second chances : a surgeon's
stories of transformation/ Donald R. Laub, M.D.

Issued in print and electronic formats.
ISBN 978-1-77041-467-9 (hardcover)
ISBN 978-1-77305-330-1 (PDF)
ISBN 978-1-77305-329-5 (ePUB)

    1. Laub, Donald R. 2. Plastic surgeons—
United States—Biography. 3. Plastic surgeons—
Developing countries—Biography. 4. Surgery,
Plastic—Developing countries.
5. Autobiographies. I. Title.

RD27.35.L38A3 2019   617.9'5092
C2018-905313-5   C2018-905314-3

PRINTING: FRIESENS   1   2   3   4   5

For my wonderful wife, Judy Laub

TABLE OF CONTENTS

BRAINS AND BRAWLS

I couldn't write the letter *g*.

I'd just finished a complicated and successful gender confirmation surgery — giving a trans man the completely functional penis he longed for using techniques I'd developed that are now the global standard. My older son assisted me in the procedure; he's a talented plastic and reconstructive surgeon, and working with him was a pleasure. My wife, all five of our grown children, and their children were thriving. So was Interplast, the medical humanitarian organization I founded in 1968 to bring free surgical care to the developing world. Since then, volunteer surgeons in association with Interplast have performed more than 200,000 life-transforming operations to correct devastating physical deformities, from cleft lips and palates to burn scars.

Though I'd recently retired as the head of the Department of Plastic & Reconstructive Surgery at Stanford University Hospital, I still had a lively and satisfying career as president of the nonprofit Gender Dysphoria Program in Palo Alto, California. I was in my mid-sixties, fit and feeling fine for a man in what I liked to think of as the early autumn of life — more like the Indian summer. All was well. I began a postoperative report to the patient, intending to write the magic words, *Surgery was successful* — but I couldn't remember how to form the letter *g*.

Soon my brain was unable to summon other letters. I couldn't walk down a hallway without bumping into walls. Then I flunked a couple of simple neurological tests. Clearly, something was wrong. "You've had a stroke," my neuropsychologist told me. "I've had a steak," I reported to my wife.

But it wasn't a steak or a stroke. It was a rare, aggressive, and lethal kind of brain cancer — intravascular central nervous system large cell lymphoma. After more than forty years as the physician, I was about to be the patient.

An extraordinarily skillful and kind team at the University of California San Francisco Medical Center deployed a new kind of "smart bomb" chemo, and after six sessions of treatment in the hospital, I recovered from a disease that has a reported survival rate of only 15 percent. That can get a man thinking.

This book is a result of those musings. It's a look back at a life in medicine, told through key moments: hard knocks, soft landings, stupid mistakes, and smart mistakes; tough choices, lucky breaks, happy coincidences, and scientific leaps; life-changing encounters with mentors, patients, colleagues, friends, and enemies. I've written this book for people who've been patients and those who care for patients; people with deep medical backgrounds and people with none. (For the latter, I've endeavored to explain medical terms and procedures in an accessible way.) It's for anyone who's interested in what makes their fellow human beings tick and how they're fixed when the ticking goes awry.

Every step of my life as a physician has been powered by the same internal forces: a deeply felt sense of duty to do good in the world; an unending appetite for interesting (i.e., difficult) cases; a love of adventure; a contrarian streak that always made me react to the word *no* with an ornery *yes*; and a dash of showmanship. Again and again, I had to take on members of the medical establishment who were quick to tell me that the things I wanted to do — deliver free surgery to the developing world; invent and improve surgical procedures that allow trans people to have the bodies they want; teach surgical interns not by the time-honored method of slowly doled-out "graduated responsibility," but through early hands-on training in the operating room — were unethical, immoral, impractical, or plain crazy. That they couldn't and shouldn't be done. At times my enthusiastic embrace of risk in the name of humane medical innovation has gotten me into big trouble. Sometimes, with the help of farsighted and forward-thinking mentors and colleagues, it's gotten big, beautiful results. And sometimes, I couldn't tell the trouble from the good results. Ultimately, the outcome has been high psychic income — the great joy that comes from saving and enriching the lives of patients, and from teaching others how it's done.

ONE

AMAZED AND SOCKLESS

I became a doctor because my father didn't, and I became a plastic and reconstructive surgeon because of a maroon Cadillac, a bunch of high school bullies who threatened to beat the crap out of me, and an embarrassing DIY tattoo.

But perhaps the path was laid even earlier.

I was almost born on December 31, 1934, at 11:38 p.m., but the doctor pushed my head back into the birth canal to await the stroke of midnight. I was unable to be brought down again by my mother's efforts, and the doctor had to extract me using forceps. I was the first baby born in Milwaukee in 1935, and my picture was in the newspaper. The pressure of the forceps accounted for a small bald area on the right side of my forehead and may, some members of my family think, be responsible for a lifetime of outside-the-box behavior. I was the second of four children, three boys and a girl. We all went to Catholic school. My father, Rudolf Laub, sold insurance, and my mother, Ella Donnersberger Laub, not only made a safe and happy home but was an energetic organizer of community projects and probably ought to have run for elected office.

Growing up in the Milwaukee suburb of Shorewood, a place with lots of elm trees and plenty of parental emphasis on education, our crew — me and the six boys I'd hung out with since kindergarten — stood out for our swagger. Or so we thought. During our freshman year at Marquette University High School, my best friend, Bill Griffith, had the habit of borrowing his father's new maroon Cadillac while his parents were at church on Tuesday evenings. He'd hotwire the car in the church parking lot by shoving a silver dollar under the ignition. Then all of us would drive around town pretending we were adults. We'd return the Cadillac just before the service let out, hoping we'd get the same parking spot. We were never caught.

One night we got cocky; we took the car right from the Griffiths' garage and drove to a football game, our school versus Whitefish Bay High School. While we were strutting around during halftime thinking we were pretty tough, some much bigger, much tougher Whitefish Bay boys picked a fight. Outmatched, we ran to take refuge in the Cadillac and locked ourselves inside. But the Whitefish Bay boys jumped up on the hood, tried to smash the windows, and put a dent in the rear fender that was detected the next morning by Dr. Griffith, Bill's father. Griff got a good licking from his mother, a tough German lady.

The seven of us dedicated ourselves to revenge, determined to beat up those Whitefish Bay guys. We taught ourselves ju-jitsu from a library book and took some rather extreme steps in our quest to toughen up. Dan Riordan cut the veins on his wrists with his hunting knife, and we drank his blood. Jack Slater fashioned some brass knuckles by pouring molten lead into a homemade plaster mold of his fist. I burned my initials, DRL, into my forearm with a cigarette in order to prove that pain could be overcome by the force of the brain — mind over matter, à la Lawrence of Arabia. I washed the wound with alcohol daily to prevent infection, and I wore a long-sleeved shirt for a couple of months so my mother couldn't see what I'd done. When the burn scabbed over and healed, my initials stood out in white. I also demonstrated the concept of mind over matter — and my toughness — by eating dirt and, I'm chagrined to recall, personal waste products. I was willing to eat shit to prove to my pals that I was a wild man.

Our self-confidence increased significantly. The next year, at the same game, we found that the menacing Whitefish Bay gang had somehow shrunken in size and ferocity. We threatened them, and they backed away before we could deliver justice.

After high school, I enrolled at Marquette University as a business major, because my father ran an insurance agency and I thought I should follow in his footsteps. I realized after two days that I hated the subject and consulted my dad. "Why did you go to business school?" he asked.

"Because you're a businessman and I was following you," I said. "What would you do if you were me?" He said he would be a doctor and told me something I'd never known — that he'd started medical school in Milwaukee but had to drop out because he couldn't afford tuition. I'd had no idea about this episode in his life, and I dearly wish now that I'd asked him more about it. The day after our talk, I switched to pre-med and instantly loved the course of study. The change also helped me make good on a rather rash promise I'd made to God in a moment of panic as a young teenager — a vow to do great good for humanity in a very particular way. I'd figured that I could keep the promise working in business by making loads of money and then giving a bunch to charity — the Robin Hood theory. But medicine would offer a more direct approach to good deeds, and the thought of becoming a healer felt much truer to my original pledge.

When I was fourteen and an enthusiastic Boy Scout, I belonged to the Wolf Pack Unit. We practiced our howls and qualified for woodsmanship badges explained in the *Boy Scout Handbook*, which was written by a naturalist I admired, Ernest Thompson Seton, the author of *Wild Animals I Have Known*. I wanted to know some wild animals, too. I thought I might get the chance when my family decided to road test a stretch of a new highway to Canadian gold country. We drove through Wisconsin and Minnesota and into Ontario, Canada, as far as a lodge at Cliff Lake, to catch walleyes and muskies. After a day of fishing and dinner at the lodge, it was still light. I hoped to hear some wolves, so I set out on a hike. I was sure I'd be fine because I had a hatchet, and I'd learned as a Boy Scout that I'd never get lost if I notched trees as I went so I could find my way back. Wolves were indeed starting to howl. Wonderful! I tried to follow the sound, and soon, despite my faithful notching, I was utterly lost, and it was dark. I tried looking for moss to indicate the north side of a tree, another Boy Scout trick, but I found none. So I built a shelter out of branches — that's what Ernest Thompson Seton would do — intending to spend the night, though I was terrified that wolves would attack. I lay down on some springy pine boughs and thought, *What are you doing? No one knows where you are, and there are wolves! Get the hell out of here.* I swore to God that if I got rescued and lived, I would become a priest.

Then I remembered another Boy Scout trick that had slipped my mind: follow a creek downhill to a bigger creek, then follow that creek to a river. This system led me back to Cliff Lake. I thought dawn was about to break, but it was only 10 o'clock when I got back to my not-nearly-worried-enough family.

Now I had a bigger problem: I was stuck with being a priest. It took me several steps to reason my way out of the deal I'd struck with God. First, I figured that only half the deal was solid — I'd lived, yes, but I hadn't been *rescued*; I'd saved myself. Yet the spirit of the bargain still seemed to require my entering the priesthood.

Even as a young child, I took seriously my relationship with the Almighty and the call to service. Consider the case of the pagan babies. When I was in sixth grade at St. Robert Catholic School, students were urged to contribute to the Pagan Baby Collection, offering money and prayers for unbaptized infants far away — Africa, I think, or maybe China. If you donated a certain amount of money, you were given the right to name a "pagan baby" in some mysterious part of the world. My classmates donated a nickel, a dime, a quarter — no baby-naming for them. I coughed up ten bucks, the entire proceeds from my summer vegetable project, earned helping in the garden of my Aunt Genny in Illinois, who had a master's degree in agriculture from a fancy eastern college. No one made me donate; I just thought it was the right thing to do. And, frankly, I'd developed a sharp yearning to be the best at whatever I tried, and that included pagan-baby salvation. My generosity entitled me to name *ten* pagan babies.

My mother wrote to my grandmother about this astonishing largesse, as well as the state of my brothers' souls. Her letter reads in part:

> Don is getting confidence very slowly but Ray
> [my younger brother] is still a big baby and
> needs to be tucked in by hand every night. Bill's
> paper route is doing a lot for him, and he hasn't
> missed another day of school . . . I urged him to
> buy himself malteds at the drug store instead of
> candy bars, and he was simply indignant: "Why,
> I can't be spending 20¢ a day on ice cream when
> I only make 60¢ — I know a kid who did that,
> and he went bankrupt — had to sell his route!"

He only contributed a quarter to the Pagan Baby Collection — whereas Don blew in $10 of his summer garden money and caused a sensation at St. Robert with the tremendous donation — ten pagan babies — and Rudy [my father] in a rage! The irony of it all is that [one of the babies] is to be named Rudolf. The Pagan Baby issue didn't bother Ray in the least. He is the King in *Sleeping Beauty* — a play they are giving. The children voted on the parts, and he said everyone wanted him to be king — he is big and jolly and has an air of superiority at school. They tell me that he can beat up all the fifth graders.

For a couple of years after the night of the wolves and the priestly promise, I went anxiously back and forth with myself about how much I still owed the Lord. Then I met a girl named Judy McCotter. Our parents knew each other, and we got together when she asked me, via my mother, to the prom at her all-girls high school, Holy Angels.

Now I really had to resolve my deal with God. I knew at sixteen that Judy, a year younger, was the one for me and decided that the honorable thing to do was to get married when we were a bit older and then help other people by doing *priest-like* work, improving lives and setting a good example. Switching from business to pre-med finally set my mind at ease. I don't know how God feels about my revised vow, but I've felt great about it ever since, regularly renewing my promise to serve. I certainly haven't felt guilty about it. In fact, I've rarely felt guilty about anything. Sad, pained, and humbled, certainly, but rarely guilty. I don't see how that would do any good for me or the people I've pledged to help. Making an error means that I've enlarged my skill and knowledge and learned what to do differently the next time.

My dad had offered to help me through Marquette Medical School by giving me $150 a month to cover various costs. He made me promise that during the academic year I wouldn't work at anything but my studies. I gratefully agreed. But almost as soon as I arrived, I was presented with the opportunity to embalm cadavers in a basement morgue for $35 a body. I considered the promise I'd made to my father and, by extension, to God, and then accepted. The $35 swayed me. I rationalized that the job was really part of my studies because it involved learning how to perform an operation on the femoral artery and vein, major blood vessels in the thigh.

I met my first cadaver during a classic Frankensteinian thunderstorm, arriving in the damp and dreary brick basement with a black bag containing all my sparkling new equipment and an anatomy book. I had studied the femoral artery and vein very carefully.

The morgue had pipes in the ceiling that contained formaldehyde under pressure, hooked up to a hose. I was to insert the hose into the cadaver's femoral artery and vein, filling the fellow's systems with formaldehyde in order to preserve the remains from bacterial degeneration. The poor body weighed about eighty-eight pounds; it belonged to a withered guy from skid row who seemed to have died of starvation.

I was about to insert the hose when I thought apprehensively, *Well, now, this guy looks like maybe he isn't dead yet.* I got out my stethoscope, listened to his heart and lungs, tried his pulse, looked in his eyes with my ophthalmoscope, and decided that he was indeed a goner. So, I started my dissection and began pouring formaldehyde into the veins. After I'd put it in about a gallon, I noticed that he'd begun to puff up. He almost looked healthy, like he was gaining weight before my eyes. I thought, *Oh my God! What if he wakes up? What am I going to do?*

I tested him again, and he was still dead. I introduced more formaldehyde, and he began to look healthier and healthier — almost robust. As I was pondering life and death and my guilt over breaking a promise to my father, the cadaver suddenly let out a loud "Ooomph!" as air from his stomach came up through the esophagus and vocal cords under the pressure of the formaldehyde. At the same time, the pressure of the fluid made his arms, which had been lying at his side, shoot straight out as if he intended to grab me. I flew back and hit the brick wall, thinking, *Oh, dear God, I'm so sorry for doing this!* I repented, quickly sewed up the cadaver, and quit the embalming business.

I would have made a lousy priest and an even worse embalmer. I was much better suited to serve as a clerk for Dr. William Frackelton, a distinguished reconstructive hand surgeon. The choice was an especially lucky one.

For starters, I was thrilled when Frackelton allowed me to assist regularly with three procedures that moved and amazed me: otoplasty — surgery to correct misshapen ears; tendon grafts to repair the soft, bandlike tissue that connects muscle to bone and thus restore mobility to shoulders, elbows, ankles, knees, and fingers; and skin grafting, replacing skin lost to burn or injury by peeling a healthy slice of skin from another part of the patient's body and carefully stitching it into place. As amazing as seeing what grafts could repair was learning that the procedure was first described in detail by the Indian surgeon Sushruta, who lived between the seventh and sixth centuries BCE. I learned how to perform these operations skillfully as a senior medical student long before they'd ordinarily come up in the curriculum. So I enjoyed a wonderful head start, racing ahead of my competitors — my fellow students.

I never did have surgery to correct my scars. That brave, stupid DIY tattoo remains a set of ever-fainter initials, their ghostly presence reminding me of a quote from the British poet William Blake, born in the eighteenth century, a maxim perfect for a fellow with a tendency to go overboard: "You never know what is enough unless you know what is more than enough." I've had to relearn that lesson quite a few times in my life.

An early example of my overzealousness came in med school. As a junior extern at the VA hospital in Milwaukee, I was on call overnight for the first time, covering all 2,000 of the hospital's patients. I was hugely excited by this important new duty, and I wanted to make sure I didn't sleep through a summons. So, I elected to sleep with the lights on whenever I was on call, usually downing a nice cup of coffee just before hitting the hay. I thought of myself as a cowboy sleeping with a loaded pistol under his pillow

Judy and I got married in 1958, while I was in medical school and she was in the middle of an internship in occupational therapy; though after we started having children, she didn't practice. What she has practiced in our fifty years of marriage, along with exemplary and extraordinary parenting, is unwavering and at times seemingly uncanny support for my healing mission. That support often came in the form of hosting in our home many, many visiting colleagues and recovering patients from around the world. It also included a stint as a successful kiwi farmer (a scheme of mine that fell to her to enact). The fact is Judy has made my work possible.

As Frackelton's fellow, I was to serve as general factotum at the 1960 annual meeting of the American Association of Plastic Surgeons, held in Milwaukee and hosted by my boss, a member of this elite society comprising the nation's top practitioners. At that meeting, I had the good fortune to witness some of the earliest public presentations of four breakthroughs that would revolutionize medicine: the first successful organ transplant — a kidney donated by a man to his identical twin — for which Joseph Murray, MD, of Brigham and Women's Hospital in Boston, would be awarded a Nobel Prize; homograft skin transplantation, which enabled badly burned patients to receive skin from another person when harvesting skin grafts from their own bodies proved impossible; craniofacial surgery — developed in France but new to the U.S. — which allowed the repair of severe facial deformities by rearranging the bones of the skull; and microsurgery that allowed the reattachment of body parts, performed using the magnification of an operating microscope, tiny instruments, and minuscule handmade needles, thinner than a human hair, fused to microsutures that enabled the connecting of blood vessels as small as five one-hundredths of an inch.

These flashy new procedures knocked my socks off, and my later introduction to gender confirmation surgery would do the same. Even now, more than six decades after medical school, the everyday marvels of my beloved specialty leave me amazed, impressed, and sockless. In those early days of training with Frackelton, I found myself tremendously touched and inspired by the puzzle and poetry of wound closure. I'd never really thought about how important and demanding the steps were, or how vital they were to a happy medical outcome, whether the wound was created by a scalpel or a boxcutter, a gunshot or a crumpled steering wheel. I wanted very much to master this art, which would require developing geometric precision; spatial imagination; thorough knowledge of the complex, multilayered anatomy of the skin and that of the rest of the body; and vigilance in preventing infection. I'd need to learn a range of psychomotor skills and learn them so deeply that they became instinctual: knowing how to clean a wound thoroughly but gently enough to preserve the cells that encourage tissue regeneration;

how to tidy a jagged wound; when to leave a wound open and when to close it; whether to use a graft or a flap; how to suture dexterously and in a way that minimizes scarring and speeds healing; and more. I found the process challenging and beautiful — and still do.

During Frackelton's presentation at the general meeting, one of my duties was to be his audiovisual aide, helping dramatically display his reconstructive skill. When, for example, he presented a case report showing ulnar (forearm) nerve palsy that had led to a claw-hand deformity, I projected a slide that showed the patient's hand with the fingers gnarled and useless. Then, as Frackelton described the surgery to repair the deformity, slides and diagrams of how it had been done appeared on the screen. Meanwhile, I guided the actual patient onto the very dark stage, both of us unseen by the audience. As soon as Frackelton was ready to show the post-op result, I switched on a spotlight over the patient's head so that only the brightly illuminated hand was visible to the audience. The patient then moved his hand to show the wonderful motion now possible. This gimmick was a big hit, and I appreciated the lesson in surgical showmanship.

An important part of the meeting was the national examination of the American Board of Plastic Surgery. These "boards" were oral and written tests for those who aspired to be certified in plastic surgery after training eighteen years post–high school. I was assigned to be the aide-de-camp to the board members, providing any kind of help they needed, from supplying cigarettes to giving directions to the bathroom. And so, I was present when the oral tests were given and then evaluated behind closed doors. In my Moleskine notebook, I jotted down — surreptitiously, I hoped — all the questions that the distinguished members of the ABPS asked the candidates. I figured these would be more or less the questions I'd be asked a few years later. This semi-secret list became my study curriculum, and, when I took the exam myself in 1971, I scored the second highest mark in the nation.

TWO

CUT TO THE CHASE

At the 1960 meeting of the American Association of Plastic Surgeons, the highest grade in the nation was earned by Robert A. Chase, MD, a young candidate who taught and practiced at Yale University. The examiners were amazed that he'd missed only one question — he'd failed to identify a pathology slide showing a rare tumor of the parotid gland, a question no one else got right either. I decided I would cast my lot with Chase at Yale, thinking that by the time I finished a five-year general surgery residency — or maybe even sooner — Chase would have established a training program specifically in plastic and reconstructive surgery, which didn't yet exist. I talked to him about this proposition at that evening's social get-together, to which both Judy and I were invited. He seemed to think that the idea was fine and was very cordial to my beautiful wife, unlike some surgeons we'd met who were dismissive of spouses. The genial New Hampshire native, exactly twelve years older than I — we had the same birthday, I would later learn — invited me to apply to the General Surgery Residency at Yale, the first step to a specialty in plastic and reconstructive surgery.

The chief of medicine at Marquette had urged me not to seek a plastic surgery residency because it was too narrow. "You have to develop your brain," he said. He and other professors advised me to take a medically oriented surgical internship like the one at Johns Hopkins. Rather than going into the operating room for each day's surgery, they explained, I'd stay on the ward solving medical, not surgical, problems; I'd have access, by way of consultation and lectures, to the top medical professors. But it seemed to me that I'd have to wait too long to get training in the actual psychomotor skills I'd need to perform surgery.

Though my heart was set on Yale and Chase, I kept an open mind and heeded my professors, also applying for internships at Johns Hopkins, Duke, Massachusetts General Hospital, and the University of Minnesota. Each of them used the medically rather than surgically oriented system of training.

When I interviewed in Minnesota, I observed an outpatient at the post-op clinic who had a little bile bag on her abdomen that drained directly from her gallbladder. She'd just come in from outside, and the bag was frozen solid. The temperature was -10°F that morning. I mentally crossed Minnesota off my list. Hopkins was fine, but I didn't feel a spark. At Duke, my jokes got a favorable response from Dr. Ken Pickrell, the reigning king of plastic surgery, whom I liked very much, but I wasn't sure about the initial focus on medicine rather than surgery.

Massachusetts General was an ordeal. I drove from Milwaukee to Boston with Joseph Geenen, a classmate and study partner with whom I'd been running nightly mock-quiz sessions. In a room with rich wood paneling on all four walls and the ceiling, haughty surgeons interrogated me on esoteric enzymes in an attempt at intimidation. But those mock quizzes stood me in good stead.

I asked to visit the ward where surgery patients were recovering and had a pleasant conversation with the chief resident, who'd been at Mass General for more than five years. He gave candid answers to my questions about the number of hours and days on duty, how involved interns and residents were in performing surgery, whether I'd have direct contact with prominent professors, and what the other interns were like. I had initially introduced myself to him as "Don Laub from Marquette University in Milwaukee, Wisconsin," but at the end of our friendly exchange, the resident said, "I'm glad to have met you. What year at Harvard are you?" I was slightly irritated, but I tried not to show it. "I'm not from Harvard; I'm from Marquette in Milwaukee."

"Oh yes, of course; I've heard of it — in the Midwest. My friend Gene Smith went out west to intern. Have you met him?"

"I don't know him," I said. "Where did he train?"

"Johns Hopkins," the resident replied. I began to

laugh, but then I realized he wasn't joking. He seriously considered Hopkins, in Baltimore, Maryland, to be "out west." With that, I knew that the rumors about Mass General's provincialism must be true.

When I got back to the motel, I learned that Joe Geenen had gotten an even rougher and more disdainful grilling than I did. Now that more than half a century has passed, I can reveal that Joe and I were so disgusted at the dismissiveness toward the Midwest displayed by the poobahs at the hospital complex that makes up Mass General (known as Ass General in some medical circles) that in the middle of the night, after downing a pitcher of martinis, we peed on the columns of Peter Bent Brigham Hospital (a.k.a. Bent Peter).

I chose Yale and became one of fifteen new surgery interns. I worked my highly competitive butt off, twelve months later earning a $200 check as co-winner of the "Best Intern" award. As usual, every time I became a little over-confident, something happened to cut me down to size. For example, under the direction of a great urology resident, we learned how to circumcise an adult male. The patient was an executive who suffered from retroperitoneal fibrosis, a relatively rare disorder that blocks the ureters, the tubes that carry urine from the kidneys to the bladder. Radiation therapy administered to alleviate his symptoms had caused scarring, which would be corrected by circumcision.

Baby boys are circumcised quickly with a device that consists of two concave stainless steel cups with very sharp edges, which are fitted in place and pressed together mechanically. But performing the procedure on a larger penis involves moving surgically around the glans, the rounded head of the penis, clamping and scissoring the skin and subcutaneous tissue, then sealing blood vessels immediately using an electrocautery machine (commonly called a Bovie after the company that manufactures it). My early training in plastic surgery allowed me to contribute postoperatively by creating a tie-over pressure dressing, covering the wound with nonstick gauze meant to provide the exact amount of pressure to allow circulation while still keeping the cauterized vessels from dripping blood. I was pretty pleased with myself.

The post-op directions to the patient were focused on prevention of bleeding. That meant no aspirin. He was to remain in bed on his back with his penis elevated a bit on a small pillow or folded towel. His wife could apply antibiotic ointment to the skin around the area of the surgery, and apply ice gently and sparingly. There could be no erection of the organ whatsoever.

Later that afternoon, I took a call from the man's wife. "Doctor, he has pain."

"Where is the pain?"

"In his head."

I responded with confidence. "That's because of the spinal anesthetic; it draws cerebrospinal fluid out of his head. How bad is it?"

"Pretty bad."

"Okay, I'll order some Tylenol with codeine. Don't give him any aspirin."

At 9 p.m., the second call came in. "Doctor, I've done everything according to your instructions. It's still hurting."

"I'll order a stronger medication. And by the way, be absolutely sure that you keep his head down, level with the body. That should fix that spinal anesthetic problem." I ordered several 50 mg Demerol tablets. I was assuming this problem was due to the anesthesia resident's inexperience.

"Doctor," the wife said, "I have very little control over him. Sometimes he has the head up."

"No! You can't have the head up even a half inch with this anesthetic. Keep it down all the time."

"But I can't control that."

"Yes, you can. Stay right beside him in bed. When he puts his head up, you push it down. Okay?"

The third call came in two hours later, to my home. "It's worse. Not only does he still have pain, but the head is bleeding!"

What? Oh! Son of a gun! I finally realized it was the head of the penis we'd been talking about. My transformation from know-it-all to chagrined idiot was instantaneous. The patient recovered nicely, and I evolved. We all had a good laugh at the post-op clinic that next week. In fact, I was offered the urology surgery training at Yale by the professor right on the spot!

I became good friends with a fellow intern, New Englander, and Yale Medical School graduate Abner Griswold Bevin, known as Biff. Biff, the lucky bastard, was way ahead of me in the one-upmanship department. He had spent a fellowship year with Chase in India, during which, he told me, he'd done a number of surgeries to restore limb function to leprosy patients. I listened enviously as

Biff described, for example, performing a finger-to-thumb reconstruction — using an index finger to replace a missing thumb — with an island pedicle flap combined with a bone graft, a rather new and fantastic operation just being introduced by Chase, who had learned it from the incredibly gifted hand surgeon Dr. J. William Littler at Valley Forge General Hospital in Pennsylvania, during a stint as an army physician. An island pedicle flap is a detached "island" of skin and subcutaneous tissue that retains its vascular supply from an underlying pedicle, or base, of blood vessels. Chase had also worked in Bengaluru, India, with Dr. Paul Brand, a British hand surgeon who pioneered the tendon transfer techniques that allow the hands and feet of patients with leprosy to function properly.

Biff touted his own abilities in long accounts that lasted until after midnight. I couldn't believe how advanced he was. But I soon understood what was going on. It was the extraordinary Chase method of teaching at work. The usual med school regimen of learning consisted of graduated responsibility, through which an intern progressively (and rather slowly) accumulates skills, earning greater and greater independence. Our mentor's unique version moved much faster. During that thumb reconstruction of Biff's, for example, Chase had been guiding the procedure. He had drawn the blue line on the skin to show Biff where to make the incision, done the dissecting of the nerve, and pointed out other important structures such as arteries — but he had allowed the intern to feel as if he'd done the entire operation himself. I figured this out because Chase would do the same with me, as he did with all the people he trained. While I worked at the cutting, Chase helped me by using his signature probe — a thin, flexible, stainless steel wand — to bring into plain view the arteries, nerves, and tendons for me to deal with according to his ongoing verbal instructions and welcome cheerleading. After three hours, Chase's students felt they'd done a world-class operation and thought they were world-class surgeons.

Chase never explicitly articulated his method of teaching, but this is what I've gleaned by observing him for more than fifty years. As students, we weren't conscious of formal teaching going on; there were no blackboards or lectures. Instruction came via attitude, energy, demonstration of vital motor skills, and joyful correction of attempts to reproduce those moves. As Chase worked, he'd describe the nature and incidence of a disease or condition, its physical and social consequence, and the alternatives for treatment. He also modeled a uniquely positive style of patient management, an example that influenced me greatly. Instead of saying, "I'm sorry, the graft didn't take. We've got to do another operation," he told the patient, "Great! You're ready for the next stage!" Chase created an oasis of benevolence that sent his students' self-esteem soaring and gave his patients a great sense of well-being.

From my arrival at Yale until this very day, my feelings about Chase have jibed with a little-known opening line of the Hippocratic Oath. Translated from ancient Greek, the oath — the earliest version of which dates from the fifth century BCE, a hundred years after the death of

Uncle Hippocrates — begins, "I swear by Apollo the physician, and Asclepius and Hygieia and Panacea and all the gods and goddesses as my witnesses, that, according to my ability and judgment, I will keep this Oath and this contract: To hold him who taught me this art equally dear to me as my parents . . ." I consider Chase to be my father in medicine.

Chase's approach to teaching was the opposite of the prevailing method of medical education at Yale. Chase wanted to build up students and make them feel as if they were great surgeons. Other professors wanted to pile on work and put us down. They adhered to a hierarchy: like medieval knights in training, we had to be pages and squires first. We interns, the pages, were assigned our day's duties first thing in the morning, and they had to be completed by 4 p.m. and okayed by a faculty member. If a task we delegated to a nurse or another staffer didn't get done, we had to do it ourselves. We might be required to do the work of a nurse, an orderly, even a custodian if that's what was needed. Turn down a job, and you were out of there. Occasionally, we had to take on the job of someone above us in the hierarchy — say, dealing with cardiac arrest on the night shift. Even if we did well, most professors were stingy with praise. But the combination of the Chase method and the Yale guild method was ultimately good for an aspiring knight of surgery.

As mere pages, we interns at Yale were subject to the ways and whims of our master teachers, not all of whom were as kindly and encouraging as Dr. Chase. The distinguished educator and practitioner Sherwin B. Nuland,

MD, known as Shep, was rather famous for being strict and brusque — some would say unnecessarily merciless — with interns. I happened to be in the room when one of these hapless underlings got pushed too far.

Late one night, Shep performed emergency surgery on a child with a bleeding ulcer. Fearing the patient would go into hypovolemic shock — a condition in which blood loss prevents the heart from pumping vigorously enough — Shep was reluctant to move the boy from the operating table to a gurney to a bed unless the transfer was done without any jolting. The orderlies were all off duty for the night. So he woke up an intern I'll call Rick, a fellow a bit tougher than the rest of us because he'd been in the navy. He was finally in bed after two straight twenty-four-hour shifts on duty, with only an hour's nap on each shift. Shep wanted Rick to help lift the patient from the operating table to the gurney. That would be all; afterward, he could go back to sleep. Too late — Rick was in the state of hyperfatigue that makes shut-eye an impossible goal. He stayed on to care for the child. The whole thing made him grumpy.

Early the next morning, resident Bernie Siegel, Rick, and I were making rounds with Dr. Nuland. The first patient was the child who'd had surgery the night before. Shep began berating and interrogating Rick. "The IV has come out, Rick. Why didn't you get here sooner to put it back in? You know you should start IVs quickly and not let the patient dehydrate. What's the result of the chest film? Have you taken the EKG? The child's hematocrit [his percentage of white blood cells] is what?

Thirty-five? I think you're making it up, Rick. It looks more like forty."

"No, Shep, it's thirty-five," Rick replied evenly.

"The temperature of this child is what? Are you up to date on the input and output? [The measure of fluids and food entering and leaving the body.] If it isn't right, you have to weigh the patient. Get the scale, now!" This was a big scale, the kind a kid had to lie on.

As Shep was barking these orders, I could tell Rick didn't like it, but he couldn't talk back; that would mean his career. He kept saying, "Yes, sir." But his face was glowing red and the veins on his neck were beginning to bulge. His hands were clenched into fists and his shoulders shook. Finally, he could stand it no longer.

Rick pounced like a cougar on his prey, grabbing Nuland's neck with both hands and pushing him against the wooden door to the room. He knocked Nuland's head against the door with a loud *bonk*, and then a reverberation, *bonkity bonk bonk*, as the door continued to bounce. He knocked Nuland against the door a second time. A third. On the third slam, he shouted, "I'm going to kill you! I'm going to kill you! I'm going to kill you!" All of this happened very quickly — but with enough time for Bernie Siegel and me to spend a nanosecond weighing just how much we hated Shep. Then Bernie pulled Rick off Shep. Neither was a small man. Both were pretty surprised at what had happened. Rick left rounds. Later that day, he was called to the office of Yale's Chief of Surgery Gustaf Lindskog, who chastised him and told him he was prohibited from ever working with Shep Nuland again.

I was assigned to work with Nuland for three months because it was believed I could get along with anyone. No mayhem ensued.

"Rick" became a successful general and cardiac surgeon in Massachusetts. Shep Nuland, having escaped attempted murder, continued to put the fear of God into interns and later made his mark as a writer. His book *How We Die: Reflections on Life's Final Chapter* won the 1994 National Book Award for nonfiction. He died in 2014 of natural causes.

My friend Biff's accounts of his fellowship year were so enticing that I signed up for Chase's next medical mission to India. But at the beginning of June 1963, a month before we were set to start the overseas year, Chase confided in me that he'd been contacted by a university on the West Coast called Stanford. "They want me to interview for Chief of Surgery," he said. At Yale, by contrast, Chase was not a chief at all but an assistant professor with no perks, no admitting privileges, no secretary, a small office next door to the morgue, and a salary of $11,000 a year. But he did have the privilege of being at Yale, an honor so great, his bosses felt, that it made up for any lack.

Chase told me that he intended to play the academic game: you get a job offer from another institution and bring that offer to the attention of your current employer; if your boss can top it, then you stay in your present happy situation but with more pay. With this outcome in mind, Chase interviewed at Stanford. The search committee found him impressive and a breath of fresh air. They also liked his groundbreaking use of 16mm motion pictures of surgical procedures as a teaching tool. He came back to Yale pleased with a nice preliminary offer. "I'm not sure I want to go to Stanford," Chase told me. "I'd be fine staying at Yale with a slightly higher salary, some beds, a research lab, an office away from the morgue, and a secretary." Chase took his nice Stanford offer to the Yale dean, who said to the young rising star, "Dr. Chase, we do not feel we have to be competitive with a tax-supported state institution like StaMford" — confusing the private California institution that would be called the Harvard of the West with the city in Connecticut.

Chase decided that he would go back to Stanford and ask for a huge salary, a huge research facility, a huge number of beds, a huge office, and secretaries galore. "They'll turn it down and all of us can retain our dignity. I'll stay here at Yale," he said to me. "You'll be fine." So he went back out to Stanford and asked for the moon and some of the stars, and they said yes to the whole celestial package. Chase took this quandary to the Yale dean who said, "Don't worry, we've saved your place for you, just as before." No raise, no perks.

The complacency and snootiness of the eastern universities was one of the factors underlying a migration of East Coast professors in the 1960s. The western salaries were attractive, and so was the feeling of being highly valued — and the elimination of the feeling that the university owned you, as well as your ideas and inventions.

Chase decided to go to Stanford and take me with him. He told me he'd try his darnedest to find some sort of position for me. The only job available was in the lab of Dr. Roy Cohn (not *that* Roy Cohn), a member of the General Surgery faculty who was about to return from a sabbatical in London where he had worked with Dr. Peter Medawar, a Nobelist whose research contributed to the discovery of how to combat the rejection phenomenon that occurred during homotransplantation (transplant between two individuals of the same species). Cohn and his Stanford colleagues were anxious to build on the work of Harvard's Joseph Murray, whom I'd heard three years earlier describing his successful kidney transplant. I was pleased at the prospect of working with Dr. Cohn, and Judy and I were excited about moving west with our three small children.

THREE

PRACTICALLY PLURIPOTENT

Dr. Cohn immediately put me to work in Stanford's experimental kidney transplantation lab. My official title was Research and Clinical Fellow in Renal Transplantation and Rehabilitation Surgery. My patients were dogs.

I didn't mind in the least. Though my tasks included scooping poop, caring for recovering animals, and occasionally getting bitten, I was also able to learn and put to use a great deal of surgical technique.

My first day on the job, in July 1963, I entered the locker room to change into scrubs and encountered an enraged man in his mid-twenties throwing his clothes into his locker and kicking it, cursing. I asked him what the matter was. We were both in our underwear. "The sonovabitch just fired me!" said Cornelis Ploeg, known as Kees (pronounced *case*). Kees had just been let go as a lab tech for a team working on preventing organ rejection, efforts that ultimately contributed to the first heart transplant at Stanford in 1968. I asked Kees a couple of questions and he gave me an earful. Before he came to Stanford, he said, he'd been at the University of Oregon, working as a lab assistant for cardiologist Albert Starr and engineer Lowell Edwards, the inventors of the first artificial heart valve, who were about to unveil an advanced version of their device. They had tested it on dogs, whose well-being was Kees's responsibility; he'd also assisted with surgery. "I was the dog's mother, father, and surgeon," Kees sputtered. "At Oregon, I placed a valve in a dog's heart on my own. Here, I'm fired because of politics." A junior lab tech wanted his job, Kees said, and had made up stories about him that got him fired.

I felt an urge, not for the first time, to rescue someone who was down and out. "Well," I said, "I'll give you a job." I marched down the hall to Chase's office and said, "I'd like to hire a lab assistant." The boss looked up over his half-glasses, widened his eyes a bit, and then said calmly, "Okay." My split-second decision, guided entirely by intuition, turned out to be a good one. This was the start of a long and happy work relationship. Kees was self-taught, highly competent, and, like me, keen to prove himself. Eventually, he would work with me to create the Stanford Primary Care Associate Program, which prepares physician assistants to practice in underserved communities.

Dr. Cohn had come back from London armed with

the latest knowledge on how to stop the rejection of transplanted organs using the immunosuppressive drug Imuran. My first assignment: to transplant a Dalmatian's kidney into a Doberman to see whether a particular chemical produced by Dalmatian kidneys would then be produced by the Doberman. (It wasn't.)

Kees and I both bicycled to the lab before dawn the day of the surgery. By 5:30 a.m., we had the patient, a feisty Doberman, shaved, fully anesthetized, on his back, and fastened to the OR table, endotracheal tube in place and ready for my incision. From the beginning, I liked the work, my colleagues, and my patients. Not only did I deepen my knowledge of basic science, but I was learning how to do a kidney transplant, which was at the time a fancy new procedure.

I was in august company at Stanford. For instance, Dr. Cohn and I were able to consult with Dr. Hugh McDevitt, the young hotshot heading the Clinical Immunology Laboratory, who was also working on the problem of organ rejection. McDevitt is best known for discovering the genes that control immune response. He determined that the human leukocyte antigen (HLA) complex — the genes that code for cell proteins that allow the immune system to recognize foreign molecules — play an important role in the rejection of donor organs. Later he would find that HLA was also vital in the preoperative matching of organ donor and recipient.

In the lab next door to ours, two cardiology residents, Bob Hurley and Bill Lauer, were getting ready to perform the first heart and lung transplant in dogs, with South

African heart surgeon Christiaan Barnard observing. Barnard would go on to perform the first human heart transplant in December 1967, using techniques developed by Stanford cardiac surgeon Norman Shumway, who had pioneered the procedure. Shumway would have beaten Barnard to the honor, but he postponed surgery because the candidate chosen wasn't well enough at the time. Shumway would do the first heart transplant in the U.S. one month after Barnard made history.

Besides arranging for me to assist Cohn on kidney transplantation, Chase graciously loaned me out to three other research projects with highly accomplished professors and physicians over the next year.

I worked with the inventor of the laser, Arthur Schawlow, and his colleagues Richard Honey and Art Vassiliadis, who were experimenting with the use of a Q-switched ruby laser to remove tattoos, first on young pigs and then on humans. This laser, containing an electrically hyperenergized synthetic-ruby rod, emits beams, controlled by the physician, that each last only nine-trillionths of a second and are at exactly the wavelength absorbed by black carbon pigment. The superfast laser is able to obliterate tattoo pigment before skin tissue had a chance to heat up, burn, and form a scar. (I think aging millennials will one day bless the Stanford team.) I hired Kees as my lab assistant for this work, too. I presented the team's findings at a national medical meeting, while the pigs stayed home with Kees.

I also worked with the distinguished educational psychologist Lee Cronbach, famous for developing ways to measure the reliability of psychological and educational tests. We created an in-service exam for plastic surgeons more meaningfully geared to the specialty than was the general surgery exam. Dr. Cronbach welcomed my ideas and the new test was given out nationwide, allowing all plastic surgery residents in training in the country to be compared to one another.

Perhaps the most intriguing investigations were in a specialty I knew almost nothing about: histology, the study of the microanatomy of cells and tissues. Another team was attempting the seemingly impossible: finding ways to heal traumatic paraplegia caused by the severing of the spinal cord. The presence of cerebrospinal fluid seemed to have something to do with preventing the nerves of a damaged spinal cord from regenerating. We experimented with placing the severed spinal cord of cats into soft tissue milieu, away from the cerebrospinal fluid that appeared to impede regeneration. I felt sure that there was some factor in the soft tissue that allowed cell regeneration. Nineteen years later, that factor would be isolated and identified as stem cells, undifferentiated cells that are *pluripotent* — not fixed as to a single line of potential development. That is, they have the ability to develop into many different types of specialized cells (say, muscle, blood, or brain) depending on what the body needs. In the last decade, scientists have made progress using stem cells to repair spinal injury, though they haven't managed to cure paraplegia. Three scientists first isolated and cultured mouse stem cells — Martin J. Evans and Matthew Kaufman at University Hospital, London, and Gail Martin at the University of

California, San Francisco (UCSF) Medical Center. Twenty years after that, physicians at UCSF would use stem cells to save my life.

During this heady period in my development as a doctor, I also asked the microsurgeon Harry Buncke, whom I had seen introduce the new field of microsurgery at the 1960 Milwaukee meeting, if I could assist with any of his reconstructive procedures. The operation that impressed me most deeply was the removal of a moderately advanced basal cell cancer one centimeter in diameter from the tip of a man's nose. First Buncke excised the cancerous tip of the nose. Then, in order to create a new tip with matching color and contour, he removed a finger-width section of the patient's forehead scalp. Leaving this flap attached to the temporal artery, he rotated it down to the nose. A temporary graft from the man's leg covered the area on the forehead from which the flap, technically a pedicle, had been taken. For twelve days this pedicle sat on the patient's nose, with the blood supply from the temporal artery bringing nourishment and circulation to what was becoming the new, growing tip. When the new tip was viable, we removed the temporary forehead graft and returned the forehead pedicle, minus the tissue that was now the new nose tip, to its original spot. To me it was a miracle. To Dr. Buncke it was just another case.

After that, Buncke invited me to help him with toe-to-thumb reconstruction and transplantation in chimpanzees, explorations vital to the refinement of microsurgery to reattach limbs. Buncke worked with his Stanford colleague

Werner Schulz, the pioneering bioengineer. He'd developed the minuscule sutures for microsurgery by coming up with a way to swage a metal needle onto human hair or the tiniest nylon strand and to operate the needle holder with a pneumatic device driven by a foot pedal. Werner also invented a penile erection device using an aortic prosthesis operated by squeezing a reservoir of saline that looked like a third testicle. One day when Buncke and I were performing microsurgery on chimps, using an operating microscope, Werner asked whether we were thirsty and would like some Coca-Cola from the machine. When we said yes, he asked how many we wanted. I said, "Well, how many can you get out of there?"

"I can get them all!" he crowed. "I invented the Coke dispenser!" I'm not sure that was entirely true, but he certainly had an impressive record as an inventor.

Whenever possible, I joined Chase in the operating room in order to deepen my skills. He taught me, for example, an interesting surgical intervention to treat dangerous pressure ulcers — bedsores — in paralyzed patients. It involved removing the bones of the lower extremities and fashioning a perfectly fitting socket cushion for the entire torso.

During that first year, I often felt pluripotent myself, as if I had the possibility of differentiating by moving into any one of several fascinating fields of exploration. But I was a clinician at heart. I missed good cases, to me the greatest source of joy and satisfaction in medicine — and by good cases, I meant the very toughest, diagnostically and surgically. Stanford was certainly a wonderland of research, but as a source of challenging clinical cases, I found it rather dull.

Luckily, a phone call in the middle of the night brought an unexpected chance to fulfill my yearning for challenging cases and make good on my immodest vow to the Lord that I would help humanity. I was about to meet the first patient who would change my life.

FOUR

PLANS A THROUGH D

Judy and I both woke on the first ring; we were used to this aspect of a physician's life. It was November 1963, and Nurse Grant was calling from the emergency room at Stanford University Hospital. "Dr. Laub," she said, "we have a bite wound — raccoon versus human. Bed number six, blood pressure 120 over 80, pulse 72. Patient has dressing on the metacarpophalangeal joint of the right thumb. He requests Dr. Chase for surgery." When someone requested Chase in the middle of the night, they often got me instead.

"We'll need an AP and lateral X-ray of the area," I said. That's a front-to-back and side view. "I'll be right in." I kissed my pregnant wife — offspring number four was due in January — dressed, threw on a lab coat, downed some instant coffee, and raced off in my gray Volkswagen Beetle. I forgot to slow down for the cop always parked in the wee hours at the off-ramp of Oregon Expressway. This wasn't the first time he'd stopped me. I told him I'd been called in for emergency surgery.

"I'll follow you in to be sure of that," he said. He came right into the nurses' station and asked, "Is the doctor really on an emergency or is it just a story for me?" I'd drilled the nurses on what to say to Palo Alto's finest if they should ever follow me in. "Oh, yes, Officer," Nurse Grant said. "We need him here. I called him to come." This wasn't a lie, but it wasn't exactly true.

"Okay. No ticket. Again."

The patient was David Werner, a naturalist and artist who was a volunteer health worker in the mountains of Sinaloa state in northwestern Mexico. He'd come to Palo Alto to raise funds for the clinic he'd opened in a remote village and was staying with friends — a physician and his wife — who had a semi-wild pet raccoon. David was trying to win over the creature with food and compassion but neither had worked.

I showed David the X-ray revealing thoroughly splintered bones. "Are you sure it was a raccoon and not a bear?" I asked. I told him that he'd need surgery to reposition and align the bones of his hand and that Dr. Chase was on his way.

Chase and I opened the wound in the operating room, further exposed the bone, and irrigated with saline to flush out raccoon-mouth bacteria. We removed the dead and contaminated tissue, cleared some periosteum (the covering of the bone), drilled holes in the bone, and put in screws and wires to hold the bones in place as they healed. Then we sutured up the soft tissue with chromic catgut, immobilized the joints above and below the fracture with a plaster cast, elevated the hand, and started David on powerful IV antibiotics.

The next afternoon, David began asking questions that were rather unusual for a post-op patient. He wanted to know a great deal about suturing, the treatment of burns, and the theory and practice of bone and tendon restoration. As David recovered and continued to pepper me with questions, I learned his story. While researching various aspects of Mexico's flora and fauna, he'd fallen in love with the country, decided to spend most of his time there, and dedicated himself to providing much-needed free basic healthcare to four small mountain villages. Though he wasn't trained as a doctor, he managed successfully by relying on the Merck manual, a handbook for physicians prepared by a large drug company, that describes the nature and treatment of virtually all medical conditions. He used the proceeds from his beautiful paintings of local birds and plants to buy supplies.

By the time David's cast came off and he began physical therapy, we'd become friends. One day, as I was examining his hand, he mentioned that in Mexico, without the help of a doctor, he'd treated three cases of tetanus — more than most physicians practicing in the U.S. will see in their careers. I was amazed. He described the great need for medical care in the area he served, where he saw cleft lips and palates galore, hernias so large they required a wheelbarrow, gunshot wounds (whenever alcohol was sufficient to catalyze disagreements), and exotic infections like leishmaniasis. Then he declared, "I'd like to learn to be a doctor." I thought for three or four seconds and said, "Okay. I'll teach you." He lit up. "But in return," I said, "I'd like to go down there with you to help out. It sounds as if you have a lot of good cases." If good cases weren't coming to me, I could go to them. I'd already started thinking globally at Yale: I'd been all set to embark on a yearlong fellowship with Chase doing reconstructive surgery in India when he got the offer from Stanford and we headed west instead of east. Now David was reviving my international dreams.

"Don," he said, "I have to return to my patients in six weeks."

"David," I said with alarm, "I can't teach you to be a physician in only six weeks!" But then I thought, *Baloney! We can do it. This guy has already treated plenty of advanced pathology by himself.* "Okay," I said. "With your huge intellect, maybe it's possible — if you apply yourself ardently." I gave David one of my white coats, covered the name *Laub* with a piece of tape and wrote *Werner* on it. "Go to the ER and observe skin suturing and extensor tendon repair" — that is, tendons of the hand, wrist, and forearm. "Tell them I sent you. I'll come down in a little while." Fifty years ago, hospital security was looser than it is today, but even by 1960s standards, I was launching a terrifically unorthodox plan. We pulled it off, though. For more than a month, David accompanied me on patient rounds and grand rounds conferences

— observing but not treating, I hasten to add. And by the time he was fully recovered, we were colleagues of a sort.

While he was my patient/student, David was working on a landmark book that would eventually sell more than two million copies in sixty languages: *Where There Is No Doctor: A Village Health Care Handbook*. He'd go on to win a 1991 MacArthur "genius" grant for his work in training grassroots community health workers. During his practical training — David called it his "emergency room apprenticeship" — the two of us had many a philosophical jam session, hashing out questions pertinent to delivering international humanitarian medicine and surgery. Is charging a fee necessary in order for a human to appreciate a medical miracle? Who should be included on trips? In places with no doctors, was it ethical for trained village health workers, highly qualified but uncertified, to deliver care? What were the best ways to respect indigenous culture? Where could we locate the money to do this kind of work? Was it ever correct to ask for the help of governments with politics we considered unsavory? We called into play law, morality, and human nature — and twenty years later, I would incorporate our conversations into the syllabus of Stanford Surgery Course 150: Principles and Practice of International Humanitarian Surgery.

David went home fully healed and full of medical knowledge. We stayed in touch, and in the spring of 1965, I drove down to Sinaloa on the west coast of Mexico in our family's new used Dodge van for a weeklong needs-assessment trip, accompanied by Kees Ploeg, his then-wife

Susan, and Judy; we left the kids with a trusted babysitter. David instructed us to turn east at a certain point, drive until the pavement ran out, then take a dirt road until it ended in a small village. After that, we traveled by mule to an even smaller village high in the mountains. David had established a home and clinic that served four communities. He called his place El Zopilote — the buzzard.

The clinic had a dirt floor, and electricity was generated by a stationary bicycle. David had helped the villagers build a simple but effective water purification system, a series of shallow pits that allowed sand to filter river water.

We learned a hell of a lot at that little clinic, starting with the way David treated abdominal discomfort in a four-year-old boy. He led the patient to a cot and had him lie down on his side. He placed a bowl of warm milk in front of his mouth. In a few minutes, an *Ascaris* tapeworm appeared in the back of the child's throat. David removed the fourteen-inch worm with forceps.

David, Kees, and I evaluated patients for a full day, assisted by Judy and Susan, and made a tentative schedule for a later surgical trip. We discussed how to maintain a sterile field, create space for a recovery room, and manage any complications since the nearest hospital was ninety-nine miles down the mountain to the west in the coastal city of Culiacán. There would be no charge for services, we decided. People didn't have much money up there anyway. We would, however, accept eggs and chickens. We'd bring all necessary medical supplies, and the visiting medical personnel would be volunteers.

Six weeks later, a highly skilled Stanford resident and clinical instructor in plastic surgery (and a heck of a banjo player), Dr. Jaroy Weber Jr., traveled to the mountain clinic as our first volunteer surgeon. Jaroy's dad was a preacher and president of the Southern Baptist Convention, and the young man felt he had received a revelation from God that he should become a surgeon traveling to all parts of the developing world.

David had gathered the patients, explained possible complications, obtained informed consent, and provided Jaroy with diagnoses and medical histories in advance of the trip. Because he was not accompanied by an anesthesiologist, Jaroy performed only procedures that could be done under local anesthesia, such as the release of burn scar contracture and small-to-medium skin grafting; cleft lip repair in a young adult using mild sedation; or scar revisions of the face, arm, leg, or abdomen. David's assistants pedaled the stationary bike to power up the clinic generator.

The second installment of the Laub-Werner project took place in November 1967, in Culiacán. This time the Stanford team was expanded to include surgeon David Dibbell, a swashbuckling Vietnam vet and former air force colonel; anesthesiologist Murray Walker; and nurses Lisa Villa and June "Brownie" Brown. David Werner had arranged for us to work at a city hospital teaming up with a respected local plastic surgeon, Jaime Galíndo. We came with a secondhand British army portable anesthesia machine, sterile supplies, vital medication, and the blessing of the governor of Sinaloa. Lisa and Brownie vigorously cleaned the operating room and surgical table — for the first time in nine years, we were told. We performed thirty-nine surgeries, most of them cleft lip and palate repair and burn scar revision. Two sisters showed up, both of whom had syndactyly — fused fingers — of the left hand. The operation to repair the condition is fairly lengthy, and we didn't have room on the schedule this time for both. They decided that the sister who was about to get married would get the surgery first, and the other would wait until our next visit. Also among the cases scheduled for a few months later was a man whose nose was bitten off by a pig when he was a baby. I had big plans for many missions to come and dreams of expanding from Mexico to Central America. But those plans and dreams hit a snag I didn't see coming.

Unbeknownst to us, our successful surgical stint in Culiacán was an embarrassment to key people in the Mexican Ministry of Health. Medical care for the poor was supposed to be provided by the government. The crowds waiting to be seen by our team made it clear that the government wasn't doing its job.

An editorial appeared in a prominent Mexico City newspaper, noting that we thought too highly of ourselves and that we were trampling on the turf of perfectly competent Mexican doctors. It even mentioned the fact that when I spoke to a local reporter in Culiacán, I had (jokingly) used the words of General Douglas MacArthur: *we shall return.*

When our team arrived for the next mission a few months later, we found that the federal government had flown in the foremost Mexican surgeon, Fernando Ortiz Monasterio, who had begun operating on the patients we'd lined up. He told us in a friendly manner, "Mexicans can take care of Mexican medical problems. I will do the cases." He had already completed four that day. The governor of Sinaloa held a lovely gathering in honor of the Stanford team, at which he offered heartfelt thanks for our wonderful work, then asked us to please leave and never come back. So much for Plan A.

I worked off my disappointment by kayaking with Dibbell on the Rio Piaxtla, which flows through one of the deepest canyons in Mexico. Shooting the rapids by moonlight cheered us up, and I began musing on how I was going to return to Culiacán and do more surgery. I came up with what I thought was a dandy Plan B: I would procure a used ship from the navy and recruit experts to teach at-risk youth from Northern California electronics, seamanship, and medical corpsman skills. We'd equip the ship with an operating room and a recovery room. Then with these young trainees — bursting with newfound esprit de corps and self-esteem — serving as crew under a qualified captain, we'd sail south with a team of volunteer physicians and ferry patients from Mexico into international waters for treatment aboard our floating clinic.

That wasn't as crazy as it sounds. When Kees, my physician's assistant, was growing up in Palo Alto, he'd been, by his own description, a juvenile delinquent. To avoid detention for his petty crimes, he'd been ordered to join the Sea Scouts, a branch of the Boy Scouts that teaches boys and girls nautical skills. He loved the training, on a decommissioned navy ship berthed in San Francisco Bay at the Palo Alto Yacht Harbor (closed in 1986 and restored to tidal marshland). After three years as a Sea Scout, he had the competency, though not the certification, to pilot a tugboat. He knew plenty of retired mariners who said they'd like to work with us as teachers. We got a grant from the Rockefeller Foundation and navigated the red tape required to obtain a beautiful ship, a 100-foot freighter built in 1943, from the Navy Reserve's mothball fleet in San Diego. Hordes of volunteer trainers in various fields offered their services. I was highly optimistic, which seems to be my default state.

Then the plan was sunk by two forces. First, a member of the Palo Alto City Council objected that our trainees, some of whom might be tough kids, would make her son and other yachters who used the harbor uncomfortable. We might have found another berth on the bay — but then the captain in charge of the reserve fleet, a raging racist, heard that we were going to be training black people as well as white, and he took back his ship. We flew to Washington, D.C., and protested up the ranks, to no avail. So much for Plan B.

Being kicked out of Sinaloa had made me feel daunted and dented but not angry; losing my navy ship because of a bigot pissed me off. I put my dream of international medical missions on the back burner until I could conjure up a Plan C. Meanwhile, my research and clinical work at Stanford was absorbing, and I was happy to be there. But I saw no great cases. Not El Zopilote or Culiacán great, anyway. Until the Latin American Mission Project (LAMP) program brought fourteen-year-old Antonio Victoria north from the Mexican border town of Mexicali to Stanford Hospital so that Chase could repair the boy's severely cleft lip and palate. Established by a group of Catholic priests-in-training from St. Patrick's Seminary, not far from Stanford, the LAMP clinic was staffed by a Mexican doctor and nurse. It served an impoverished neighborhood, charging a minimal fee for medical services — less than twenty-five cents a visit — so that those seeking help could maintain their dignity and not feel like charity cases.

Where Antonio's lip should have been, there was instead a catastrophic triangular hole revealing moist tissue beneath. Because of this abnormality, the boy had never gone to school, and he had few friends.

As a fetus develops, key parts of the head and face first form separately and then gradually merge, fusing at the philtrum, the groove on the upper lip. In some babies, however, those parts don't meet completely because of genetics or environmental factors or both. The result is a fissure in the upper lip and palate — the roof of the mouth — called a cleft. That cleft can distort the teeth, gums, and facial bones, making it difficult for the child to eat, speak, and, sometimes, hear.

The incidence of cleft palate was especially high in the Mexicali Valley, experts conjectured, because of substandard nutrition and advanced paternal age; research also suggested that pesticides used in the fields might have contributed to the problem. In the U.S., where these deformities occur in one out of every 600 to 1,500 births, they're repaired immediately. But in impoverished and underserved Latin American communities, reparative surgery for afflicted children and adults was either inaccessible or unaffordable.

Chase called me in to take a look at the boy. We felt for him, of course, as human beings and fathers. As a scientist, however, Chase also saw in Antonio a rich research opportunity. He could help us study muscle development, the enzymes that control bone growth, and the speech problems caused by significant facial deformity. The proposed research certainly sounded interesting. But I would soon have other ideas.

I scrubbed in and played a minor role in the three relatively brief operations, performed with textbook precision, that dramatically and permanently improved Antonio's face and future. After a trouble-free recuperation with a welcoming foster family, the teenager went back to Mexicali with a slight, manly scar on his lip, movie-star handsome.

Antonio's metamorphosis reignited the delight I'd taken in cleft lip and palate repair in Culiacán. "I wish I could take on more cases like Antonio's," I said to my boss rather wistfully. "But we have so few here."

Chase appointed me chief of Plastic & Reconstructive Surgery at Stanford University of Medicine. The title was terrific, though there was no official PRS division yet. I was immersed in my daily work, but Antonio's transformation remained on my mind. One day in 1968, I called Phil Collins, the bilingual American who served as LAMP's community organizer in Mexicali, just to see how the boy was doing. "Fine," Phil said. "More than fine. He's in school for the first time, and he already has lots of guy friends and a girlfriend. What a change in that boy!" I was struck by how quickly cleft lip and palate repair had allowed him to trade isolation and sorrow for a happy, productive life.

"Are there any more cleft lip cases in the Mexicali area?" I asked Phil.

"Hundreds!" he said. I couldn't wait to tell my boss. Within a week, we were headed for Mexicali, a place teeming with "good cases," kids we might be able to bring up to Stanford for life-changing surgery like Antonio Victoria's.

I had no idea that this adventure in Mexicali would be the first of 159 volunteer surgical trips all over the world. All I knew was that I wanted to help these people waiting patiently on benches outside the clinic and that it was hot as hell — 110 degrees by 10 a.m. "Don't touch anything metal outside after nine in the morning," we'd been warned by Phil, a former insurance agent who lived in Mexico thanks to the federal witness protection program; he'd testified against the mob in Chicago. "You'll give yourself a first-degree burn."

Rain is rare in dusty Mexicali; its cotton, alfalfa, and sorghum fields are irrigated by the same system that makes California's Imperial Valley bloom. But the previous evening, hours before Chase and I arrived, rain came for the first time in three years, a downpour so hard we couldn't drive our car to the clinic building, a converted house in a neighborhood with dirt streets. We had to get out and walk barefoot through mud two inches deep. We spent the night at the home of Phil and his Mexican wife, Luz, not far from the clinic; I slept on a cot, and Chase bunked on Phil's pool table.

By morning the streets were dry. Nearby stock-yards, where cattle were fattened on Mexicali grasses, emitted a slight lingering stink. The fighting cocks that someone kept in a pen behind the clinic were crowing. Phil had canvassed the neighborhood to gather people needing the help of a reconstructive surgeon. Most of the patients waiting were children, many with unre-paired cleft lips and palates, and some who had been badly burned, usually from getting too close to an open cooking fire or kerosene stove or accidentally tipping over boiling pots. Without the right treatment, the burns had healed improperly, leaving disfiguring or immobilizing scars — thickened, ropey ripples of flesh that marred their faces or contracted to fuse their chins to their chests or their arms to their sides. If medical care were available, such scars could be released and the skin repaired with skin flaps or grafts. A relatively brief procedure could transform a face or restore mobility. But the people waiting at the clinic had, until now, no chance of receiving such treatment.

In Mexico back then — and elsewhere in the develop-ing world, I would learn, except in the most cosmopol-itan cities — a child or adult with a deformity was often doomed to life as a pariah. Though some communities embraced the disfigured, too many regarded the cleft lip or palate or the phantom-of-the-opera burn scar not as accidents or randomly distributed flaws but as a judgment from God, punishment for some hidden sin. It wasn't unusual for children with facial anomalies to be kept out of school, so that they grew up illiterate, hard to employ, and miserably isolated. Nine-year-old Eugenio Lara, the very first person I evaluated in Mexicali, was on his way to becoming one of those outcasts. Waiting with his grandmother in the searing morning sunlight, Eugenio wore a brown paper bag over his head, with two holes cut out so he could see. Through an interpreter, I gently asked the grandmother what the bag was for. "He has a burn scar on his face, and it pulls down his eye," she said. "The other kids make fun of him. He is hiding."

Eugenio, we learned, was epileptic. He was injured when he had a seizure and fell into the cooking fire on the floor of his family's house, little more than a hut. When I lifted the bag he was wearing, I saw that the tug of a contracted burn scar under his eye had turned the lower eyelid inside out, a condition called an ectropion. Chase told me that if the eyelid remained exposed to the wind and dust of the desert, Eugenio would eventually end up with keratitis, an inflamed cornea, a condition that if left untreated could lead to blindness. We talked a great deal about the social damage the ectropion caused Eugenio — that paper bag had startled both of us — and how we should proceed. We agreed that a full-thickness skin graft harvested from the inside of his elbow would be effective. And a small cartilage graft from the tip of the external ear, another beautiful donor site, would help keep the eyelid propped up.

I was powerfully drawn to the idea of helping this boy, who would turn out to be the catalyst for Plan D. I thought for a *momentito* and said, "Eugenio could come to Stanford, and we could do the surgery there."

"We could," said Dr. Chase.

"But if I made an arrangement with a local hospital, I could come down with the right equipment and do this case and lots of others."

"Yes, you could."

I looked at the list of patients waiting to be seen — the many children with cleft lips and palates, a girl with a burn scar contracture that fused her arm to her torso, a man with a large basal cell tumor of the nose. My thoughts raced. *We could hold a clinic on weekends or maybe monthly. We have connections through LAMP to doctors down here who could gather needy patients. We could do fundraising in the States. We could teach medical students from both countries.* I felt a sudden coalescence of all my previous training and experience into a clear career path. But could it work? I'd already been kicked out of Mexico once.

In consultation with Chase, I devised a collaborative model for a project that would combine personnel from Mexicali and Stanford into one team. Then, with some trepidation, I talked to doctors belonging to the Colegio Médico, the medical society, of Baja California, the Mexican state where Mexicali is located. They were enthusiastic. So was the local Rotary Club. Next, I got the permission of state officials. My big worry was the central government — the health ministry so offended by my work in Sinaloa state. But it turned out that they didn't care what happened in the northern Baja California state; they seemed to feel that it was so close to the border it was practically American anyway.

We signed an agreement, a *convenio,* with the governor of Baja California, LAMP, the Mexicali Rotary Club, and the Colegio Médico, stating that we would perform surgeries for no charge to patients at the local *hospital civil,* bringing all equipment, supplies, and medications — everything from antibiotics to gowns, drapes, and gloves. We would provide an anesthesiologist from Stanford, as well as a speech therapist, dentist, and orthodontist. Postoperative care would be handled by local surgeons, and a physician assistant from Stanford would stay on-site for two weeks after every trip to oversee follow-up care. We would train Mexican medical professionals. Each member of the Mexicali plastic and reconstructive team would be paired with their counterpart at Stanford, and Mexicali would, in time, become a second Stanford practice site.

When I got home from Mexicali, I hit up local service organizations for small donations, and Judy held a fundraising walkathon. Four months later, I repaired Eugenio's face at the *hospital civil* in Mexicali, a twenty-eight-bed facility that shared a building with the local jail. He was able to discard that paper bag forever, and on the trip after that, Eugenio came to the hospital with his grandmother, shook my hand, thanked me, and told me that he was in school and had friends.

Over the next three years, I would treat hundreds of

patients in Mexicali and revive my dream of bringing surgical care to Central America and beyond. Eugenio was the patient who pushed me to begin making those dreams a reality. But another boy I met on that first trip to Mexicali inspired a new level of commitment to what started as the Mexico Medical Project and became Interplast. His name was Salvador, and he changed my life.

FIVE

THE PERFECT SMILE

Nine-year-old Salvador seemed like just the kind of kid we could fix. His otherwise lovely face was marred by a bilateral cleft in his upper lip, two gaping holes in a twist of flesh with crooked teeth poking through like tiny tusks. His nose was flattened. Teased and tormented by the kids in his neighborhood — as well as too many of the adults — he'd spent most of his seven years inside his family's small concrete-block house in Mexicali, surrounded by the inhospitable Sonoran Desert.

Chase and I felt sure we could give Salvador a new life with a single surgery to fix his fissured face. His mother, Julia Anita, was ecstatic. She'd heard from the clinic that American doctors were coming, and she was convinced they could help her son live a normal life. Now that conviction had been corroborated by two surgeons.

But then there was trouble. During a thorough physical exam, we detected a heart murmur that suggested a defective valve. "Your son has a heart problem," we told Julia Anita. "We can't operate on him. It would be too dangerous." She was devastated. But she wasn't ready to take no for an answer. Several weeks after my first trip to Mexicali in 1968, I returned with supplies, equipment, and a volunteer medical team from Stanford to perform surgery in a small community hospital with the permission we had obtained from the state government and the local medical society. Julia Anita and Salvador were back in the line of patients to be assessed for future surgery.

This time we had a pediatrician with us. The answer was the same: without a cardiac catheterization, a sophisticated diagnostic procedure in which a long, thin tube is inserted into an artery or vein and threaded through blood vessels to the heart, corrective surgery on Salvador's face was too risky. We didn't feel comfortable doing a catheterization at the small local hospital. We could bring Salvador to Stanford, but that would divert scarce funds that could otherwise repair the lives of many other children.

Salvador's mother refused to give up. In 1971, she brought her son back for a third try at surgery. Three years had passed since I'd first examined the boy. By now, our volunteer team had grown to comprise a pediatrician, two anesthesiologists, four plastic surgeons, an American and a Mexican nurse, and two Mexican interns doing required national service.

The pediatrician examining Salvador furrowed his brow as his stethoscope amplified the *whoosh, whoosh, whoosh* of the heart murmur. To his expert ears, it sounded like an atrial septal defect, a hole in the wall of tissue separating the top two chambers of the heart. He shook his head. Yet again, the answer was "We're so sorry, but no surgery."

Julia Anita pleaded with us. "Doctors, Salvador has only one chance for a normal life. He has been turned down twice. Without surgery, he is nothing. Other children call him The Monster. The operation is worth the risk! Please, *please*, doctors, give him the chance!"

Our team passionately discussed the pros and cons of the case. We talked over the ever-present risk of complications, the methods we could use to minimize problems, the life that awaited Salvador if we didn't take a risk, the grim outcome for him and for us if that risk didn't pay off. Should we put our reputations on the line to help a mother begging us to reprogram her son's doomed future? *What is God's plan here?* I wondered. Back and forth we went. Salvador was evaluated even more carefully and provisionally diagnosed with an atrial septal defect. The condition did pose a surgical risk, but the treatment team concurred that the risk was small — perhaps a 2 percent chance of complications. I was the trip chief, so I made the final decision. We would give Salvador his shot at a happy life.

The equipment we'd brought with us from Stanford was already unpacked and our instruments sterilized. We sterilized them again. We set up the electrocardiogram, the only monitoring device we had in the late '60s; it tracked blood pressure and pulse. The pO_2 meter, which measures oxygen levels in the blood, and the pCO_2 monitor, which ensures that a patient is being ventilated correctly, hadn't been invented yet.

We were ready for a backup blood transfusion if necessary. We checked and rechecked Salvador's lab work.

Salvador walked into the OR on his own and hopped up onto the table. He trusted us completely because his mother had told him he should. Induction of anesthesia, the riskiest event in Salvador's life thus far, was absolutely routine. The two anesthesiologists, both superior and soon to be nationally acclaimed, saw and heard no indication of danger. We all approached the case with enthusiasm. "Let's go," I said.

I'd chosen Terry Knapp, MD, a Stanford colleague, as the lead surgeon for Salvador's procedure, the third case on a blazing hot Saturday. Terry was turning out to be larger than life in several spheres: his surgical technique and organizational abilities were excellent; he had a drive for self-improvement; he was intense and funny. He would go on to cofound the Collagen Corporation while he was still a resident at Stanford, and he's since become a notable physician-entrepreneur.

"Position the head, Terry," I instructed. I asked our team nurse, Jeanie Roe, to cleanse the skin and place the sterile drapes. Using a sharpened Q-tip dipped in methylene blue dye, Terry drew the blue lines showing where we'd cut into Salvador's knotted flesh, then stretch, smooth, and stitch the skin to create a normal lip. Terry and I remeasured the geometric pattern of the incision to the half millimeter.

We explained the plan to the observers in the room — medical professionals from Mexico, including our sponsoring local physicians, Dr. Benjamín Garza Canales and Dr. Miguel Angel Rolón, who were monitoring us for their medical society, checking the quality of our work, as well as students from both countries — and we taped a diagram on the wall of the operating room.

Fixing the twisted skin, muscles, and mucous membranes of a cleft involves loosening and freeing tissues by cutting into the three layers and recruiting these existing resources to reconstruct an anatomically normal lip. Most important is repairing the muscle, which, as it heals, will pull the cleft together to bring teeth, underlying tissues, and skin into a normal anatomic position. The art is in freeing up tissue while maintaining the blood supply, which is necessary for healing and growing. In a later procedure, we'd fix the characteristically flattened nose using the patient's own cartilage as the building block of a new projecting tip.

"Sponges, please. Terry, make the skin incision with your smallest scalpel." I gently put the plastic surgery hooks on the little flaps of skin created by the incision. "Wider yet, please, to free up the muscles," I said. "Be just as careful as the Sierra Club." Terry knew I meant the surgical version of the nature lover's motto *take only pictures, leave only footprints*: do no harm, be gentle and fine, leave no trace of surgical trauma.

Terry flopped open the whole lip and loosened all

the tissue of the cheek, almost to the parotid glands in front of the ears. Now the entire face was open, a mask of red tissue that looked like a battlefield injury. The jigsaw puzzle was set for reassembly. "Okay, everything is ready for the reconstruction," I said. Terry prepared to place the initial sutures. The foundation of a new construction like this one is the periosteum, the covering of the dental arches — the upper jaw bone. Then come the mucosa, the muscle, and the skin. Each layer is sutured separately. The repaired muscle works to create a sort of ongoing orthodonture. When the lip is cleft, the muscle is split, and the brain signals each side separately, so they pull apart. After the muscle is fixed, the brain sends a different signal, and the muscle pulls in the bones of the jaw, straightening the teeth into the proper position.

Terry asked the Mexican scrub nurse for a 4-0 chromic suture. "*Cuatro-cero crómico, por favor.*" Everything was going great. I thought about how much the organization had grown in just three years. We'd started medical missions to Guatemala and Honduras; Stanford residents were doing rotations there and in Mexico with professors from those countries; and we were participating in conferences where North American and Central American physicians could exchange ideas. Things were going so well, I thought, that we should expand all over the world. I was picturing a radiantly rosy future when one of the anesthesiologists suddenly spoke: "People, we have no pulse."

In the operating room, the conditioned response to that information is action. I checked the child's airway.

Was the endotracheal tube in place? Was it kinked, clogged, or full of blood? Was the child's blood blue? Was the carotid artery pulsing? We listened for heart sounds, checking to make sure oxygen was flowing into his lungs and that there were no mechanical problems with the machine supplying oxygen. The checklist was completed with staccato timing in ten seconds. Everything was in order. I started external massage, pushing down on the chest to squeeze blood in and out of the heart.

"Is there any electric action?" I asked our anesthesiologist. "Is there fibrillation?"

"No!" he called. "Flatline. Flatline. Flatline."

"Okay, stimulate with intracardiac epinephrine and give bicarbonate to reverse acidosis. Let's give a swift blow to the chest to stimulate the first heartbeat." I remember praying, *Dear God, if this child lives, I will be good the rest of my days. I'll devote myself entirely to the well-being of others. Oh, shit.* It was an amen of a sort. As I worked on Salvador, I thought, *Why did I go out of the way to take chances? Why did I come to Mexico? Why did I ever become a doctor in the first place? Oh, shit. Why is this happening? How can we save this child's life? What could I have done differently? Oh, this is awful, awful, awful. But let's do whatever is needed now . . . What would I say to his mother? What would I say to my mother? How could I get out of jail in a foreign country?*

My mind was going a thousand miles an hour. Then the anguish I felt because a child might die was superseded by the need to keep cool and form a plan instantly.

Focus, I said to myself. *What resources do we have here that can save this situation?*

None, it turned out.

Less than half an hour later, Salvador had been removed to the hospital morgue. Terry and I were in the waiting room with Dr. Garza Canales, our mission coordinator Phil, and Salvador's mother. I looked at the wall, at the floor, and then into Julia Anita's eyes, and took a deep breath. *"Señora, tuvimos problemas, complicaciones muy graves. No hemos tenido éxito; Salvador ha muerto."* We had problems, serious complications. We did not succeed; Salvador has died.

Her tears were explosive. I stood with her in sorrow, surrealistically aware of incidentals — trash on the hallway floor, the smell of excrement from the ward room where six dirty, unshaven men were struggling with their own wounds, a flying insect, the pure blue of the sky glimpsed through an open door.

Then Salvador's mother looked at me and spoke quietly. Dr. Garza Canales translated her sad, sweet speech. "You needn't be so upset, doctor. You and your colleagues did your job as well as you could. Salvador was given his chance, and he won, because his lip is finally repaired, and he will see God with a perfect smile."

This woman has so much wisdom and grace despite her pain, I thought. And then, half a second later, *Oh my God! His lip isn't repaired. His face is a mess!*

Terry Knapp had the same realization simultaneously and jammed his elbow into my ribs. Julia Anita expected to have an open coffin at Salvador's funeral so that she and God and all her neighbors could appreciate Salvador's beautiful and complete face. We had to make that happen.

But operating on dead bodies is against the law in both Mexico and the U.S.; doing so is considered mutilation. Again, we conferred as a team, discussing the situation in English and Spanish. The response was unanimous. Everyone said some version of the same thing: "This mother deserves the best-looking face we can make. The patient is more important than the law. Let's go!" This decision could have gotten us in real trouble; it could have created an international scandal. But that was a risk we felt obligated to accept. Salvador's body was retrieved from the morgue. As I walked back to the operating room, I went through the next moves in my mind: *clean Salvador's face, put on drapes, recheck the pattern of the flap. We won't need anesthesia; we won't need sponges; there will be no bleeding.*

In thirty minutes, we were all satisfied. One of the young residents, Howard Holderness, said he would buy a coffin and attend the boy's funeral as our representative.

At dawn on Sunday, the rest of the team was back at work in the hospital performing surgery to fix other children's cleft lips. There was no sound except for the sigh of the steam autoclave sterilizing instruments and the clicking of surgical needle holders, the scissorlike tools that allow a surgeon to manipulate a suturing needle. At 9 a.m., we looked out the open window, and our minds soared through the clearest of blue skies to the neighborhood church so that we could all be there in spirit as Julia Anita got her first look at Salvador's new face.

The team completed eleven cleft lip and palate reconstructions that weekend, ten of them rather dramatic rehabilitative successes. The parents' joyful tears when they viewed the now-normal faces of ten of those children gave us enough psychic income for another year of volunteer work — and then we got a bittersweet bonus. Howard returned from Salvador's funeral and told us what had happened. When Julia Anita saw Salvador's face, she exclaimed, "He is beautiful! Look what you have done!" And through her tears, her face was joyfully illuminated by her own perfect smile.

As we packed up for the trip north, I was deeply mourning Salvador. The boy's death was devastating — an abyssal experience. Yet somewhere within me, I felt a rush of energy that seemed to contain the possibility of sorrow's opposite. I felt compelled — committed — to do more. I envisioned a clear path, a grand plan for providing surgery to the disadvantaged all over the world, while teaching men and women who wanted to be surgeons how to combine skill and compassion in order to spread joy.

On Monday, back at work, I experienced culture shock. My assistant ran through all my messages. A patient who'd had cosmetic surgery was a bit uncomfortable; she needed me to call her immediately. My insurance saleswoman, my CPA, and my attorney all wanted me to give them a buzz as soon as possible. Someone had a great investment opportunity for me and wanted me to get in touch quickly; someone in administration said I'd filled out a form incorrectly, and I had to get back to him right away. My thoughts were still with Salvador. After what had happened in Mexicali, I felt that these people were all ridiculous, and answering their messages was unimportant.

And then I had an idea. I did something I'd never done before: I called back each of these people and said, "I'm going to tell you about a great project, and I'm sure you'll want to help. There's a 1,000 percent return on investment." Then I told each of them the story of Salvador and asked them to donate generously to our volunteer surgical missions to Mexicali. To my surprise, all of them — the patient, the CPA, the administrator, the insurance woman, everyone — said yes! Furthermore, they all thanked me for giving them a chance to do good in the world.

That was when the organization that would be called Interplast went into turbo-drive. I tithed my time: for the next eighteen years, I gave 10 percent of my efforts to building the international enterprise. And in the fifty years of the organization's existence, the volunteer doctors of Interplast (now called ReSurge International) — physicians from all over the globe — have delivered more than $5 billion in medical services in fifteen countries on five continents, at no cost to the patients.

And all of this extraordinary work was propelled by David Werner's example, Eugenio's urgent need, and brave Salvador's tragic death, a catastrophe that strengthened my sense of mission, gave the project tremendous momentum, and propelled me to reach out for support in a way that was new to me.

SIX

THE RIGHT THING

Over the course of my career, I've often caught myself saying, "You know, that patient changed my life." In truth, everyone I treated in more than four decades as a surgeon has altered me for the good in ways large and small, as I altered them. But after a great deal of thought, I've managed to narrow that vast field to four — four patients who truly transformed my career path, my sureness of purpose, my skills, and my heart; four people who sparked actions on my part that ultimately affected hundreds of thousands of others all over the globe. David Werner, the genius rural health worker who awakened my passion for international humanitarian medical service, was one of them. Eugenio, who motivated me to get my grand plan off the ground, was another. And of course, there was Salvador, the patient who left such a huge impression on all of us.

The fourth person who changed my life forever was Ella.

David Dibbell, now my chief resident, knew how to hook me. He called me in for a consultation during our weekly clinic. "Don," he said, "this is not a good case. This is a *great* case. The diagnosis is transsexualism. The patient was born the wrong sex and wants a surgical change. Go into the exam room and see for yourself."

It was 1968, the same year in which I'd met Salvador and Eugenio for the first time. I am a Catholic from the Midwest; changing what God made goes against many of my beliefs. The one thing that can overrule my religious beliefs is my fervent desire to do the right thing. And if this diagnosis was correct, it was clear to me what the right thing to do would be. "I do love a great case," I said.

I entered the exam room and introduced myself to a beautiful woman wearing a hospital gown — I'll call her Ella — and commenced a thorough physical exam, from top to bottom. Ella had long, blonde hair in loose curls; her makeup was impeccable, and her voice had an appealing Lauren Bacall rasp.

"Dr. Laub," Ella said as I tapped and palpated, "are you familiar with transsexualism?"

My answer was "Not fully." That was a know-it-all young doctor's way of saying, "I just heard about it for the first time two minutes ago."

"Have you read Dr. Harry Benjamin's book, *The Transsexual Phenomenon*?"

"I'm afraid I haven't," I said. *Who the hell is Harry Benjamin?* I thought.

"Dr. Benjamin sent me here to Stanford."

As I examined the lovely Ella, I soon discovered generous genitalia, undeniably male. *Oh my God,* I thought. *I thought I knew everything there is to know about plastic surgery. I can close any wound ever created — and I've never heard of this diagnosis until today. Not only that, but I made a mistake about the patient's sex!* I asked Ella to dress, left the exam room, and hailed Dibbell.

"Isn't this terrific?" he said. "Let's call Harry Benjamin in New York this afternoon! He's the guy who knows everything about transsexualism." That diagnostic term is out of date, and transsexual people are now considered part of the broader transgender continuum. But fifty years ago, all of this was new to us. "Are you in?" Dibbell asked. I was. We told Ella, who was seeking surgery to complete her physical transition, that we'd look into her case.

During our lunch hour that day we called Dr. Benjamin. An endocrinologist who'd come to New York from Berlin in 1910, Harry Benjamin was a pioneering physician, scientist, and educator, widely regarded as a kind, respectful human being and a brilliant, innovative practitioner. He'd embraced as his specialty what would eventually come to be known as gender dysphoria — the condition of a person's gender identity being different from the one assigned based on anatomy and hormones — and he was an early advocate of what we then called sex-change surgery. Benjamin, who died in

1986, was a tireless and compassionate advocate for the transgender community. We had a lot to learn from him.

"Yes, this is a legitimate condition," Dr. Benjamin told us that day. "The brain is separated functionally from the body, in that one is male and the other female — for example, a male body and female behavior residing in the brain. It occurs right from birth. The cause is not yet clarified, but it is real." Benjamin's staunch, and at the time revolutionary, insistence that gender dysphoria is a medical problem, not a mental disorder, has been accepted by most, though not all, scientists and physicians. The condition's precise biological causes have yet to be discovered and are still being investigated by neuroscientists doing promising brain studies. According to today's figures, about a million and a half Americans experience gender dysphoria. "I can send you more patients," Benjamin said that day, "at my expense."

We eagerly assented, and within a month we had two more male-to-female patients lined up besides Ella. Benjamin had already started them all on the hormone estrogen, and they planned to get breast implants. They needed us to swap their functioning penises for functioning vaginas.

Roughly one in 30,000 adults who were assigned male at birth and one in 100,000 adults who were assigned female at birth seek what was once called sex-change surgery, then sex reassignment surgery. These days I prefer the term "gender confirmation surgery" or "gender-affirming surgery," which are more exact and humane. Some people with gender dysphoria prefer not to undergo surgery at all; many of them instead choose a hormonal transition.

In preparation for Ella's surgery, I immersed myself in the history of the field. The earliest operations, performed by European doctors in the 1930s, were crude and only sporadically successful. The procedures became more refined in the late 1940s and included the administration of the appropriate hormones. Christine Jorgensen, an American former GI who had been assigned male at birth, made big news in 1952 after transitioning with the help of Danish surgeons; Harry Benjamin oversaw Jorgensen's additional surgery in the U.S. In the 1960s, the French gynecologist Dr. Georges Burou, practicing in Casablanca, Morocco, pioneered a procedure that created a vagina from an inverted penis. In the U.S., the 1960s brought a boom in funding for medical research — but not for programs studying and treating "transsexuality," a controversial specialty that wasn't supported by the American Medical Association or government health agencies. The work of Benjamin and Milton T. Edgerton, who founded the first U.S. university-based transsexual surgery clinic at Johns Hopkins in 1965, was initially funded by a wealthy trans man, Reed Erickson. The first person to undergo gender confirmation surgery in the U.S., trans woman Phyllis Wilson, had to get permission from a Baltimore court before going under the knife.

At Hopkins, Edgerton formed a multidisciplinary team that included not only plastic surgeons and anesthesiologists but also a psychiatrist, urologist, gynecologist, theologian, social worker, and an attorney. Following his

lead, Stanford psychiatrist Norman Fisk and I assembled
our own interdisciplinary team. From the beginning, we
obtained informed consent with an attorney as witness,
present when we explained the surgery and its risks to the
patient; he would be our legal counsel if there were any
problems. Fisk and I visited every place in the world where
gender surgery was being done, and Harry Benjamin came
to Stanford to lecture and attend grand rounds.

Back then, gender confirmation surgery was riskier
sociologically and politically than medically, but it was an
operation new to us, and so as we thoroughly prepared,
I thought of the maxim about taking chances that I'd
learned early in my medical training from a veteran professor: don't put your balls on the chopping block unless
you're willing to have them chopped off; that's how sure
you should be of your decisions. It seemed extremely apt
in this case. (And looking back, I can see why female med
students rolled their eyes at this advice.)

Ella's procedure, the first gender reassignment surgery in California, was scheduled for November 1968.
The three-and-a-half-hour operation involved forming
a vaginal space between the rectum and the bladder and
then using the procedure developed by Georges Burou
in Casablanca to invert the penis, essentially turning it
inside out to create a vagina, with the scrotum altered to
serve as labia. The operation preserved the nerves that
allow sexual sensitivity. I was the head surgeon, and
things went well. Ella was pleased.

And then she sued me.

I was away on a Mexico Medical Project trip to Mexicali

when she experienced some minor bleeding on the ninth day after her surgery. The problem was handled quickly and competently by my resident surgeon, who'd participated in her procedure. Ella remained happy with her transformation. But a misguided friend had told her that if she filed a lawsuit, the surgeon wouldn't send a bill, and she'd get her surgery for free. So, I was served.

I was devastated and spent many nights awake at 3 a.m., thinking about how to deal with this terrible blow. No one had ever sued me before. The strategy I came up with was continuing to do gender confirmation surgery, building up experience so that by the time the lawsuit came to court, I would be the most qualified expert witness in the world.

As it happened, the lawsuit never did go forward. Ella failed to appear for a deposition and apparently abandoned this financial tactic. A year later, she contacted me and suggested we write a book together as if she'd never launched the distressing adversarial action. I politely declined, but I stuck with my late-night strategy of working to become an expert, in both the operating room and the courtroom. Over time, I would perform 900 surgeries for transsexual patients, including 250 complete sex changes in either direction. And I would testify at the trial of the world's worst — and most lethal — "sex-change doctor." More about that later.

Transsexualism as a diagnosis was included in the American Psychiatric Association's *Diagnostic and Statistical Manual of Mental Disorders* in 1980 — *DSM-III*, the third volume of the highly regarded professional resource first published in 1952 and updated every decade or so. No mention was made of transsexualism in any volume until *DSM-III*, where it was located under "Disorders Usually First Evident in Infancy, Childhood, or Adolescence." The term gender identity disorder replaced transsexualism in the 1994 *DSM-IV*. This diagnosis was assigned to patients who fulfilled a short list of signs and symptoms: those who had the anatomy, hormonal secretions, and phenotype of one sex but identified as the opposite sex and behaved according to that belief.

Some psychiatrists were firmly convinced that gender dysphoria was indeed a disorder, a mental illness, and one that couldn't be successfully treated by changing the body through surgery. Instead, they insisted, the right thing to do was to use behavioral therapy to adjust the brain to match the body the patient was born with. This behavioral modification sometimes included aversion "therapy" — the patient received a shock if they exhibited behavior incompatible with the sex assigned at birth.

Finally, in the 2013 *DSM-5*, gender identity disorder was replaced by the designation gender dysphoria, coined by my colleague Norman Fisk. The term is especially apt because, as Nicholas M. Teich notes in his excellent book *Transgender 101*, it "emphasizes the anguish that results when a person's psychological sex, or gender, does not match his or her physiological sex, or body."

Any moral doubts I had about gender confirmation surgery had evaporated during that first telephone conversation with Dr. Benjamin in 1968. These patients felt tormented, and I could help eliminate their anguish through surgery, a transformation as powerful as the ones our Mexican Medical Project was bringing to children and adults with cleft lips, burns, and other deformities. Still, I wanted to know what Catholic theologians had to say about gender confirmation surgery. I consulted a Jesuit priest, Father Robert O' Reilly, an expert on canon law. He told me that two areas of canon law covered gender confirmation surgery. The principle of the destiny of parts, he explained, says that each part of the body has a purpose and you must not obliterate that part because you obliterate God's intended purpose. But the doctrine of the whole says that a person consists of a mind and a body, and if they're divergent, one or the other may be changed in order to make the person whole. Science had failed at changing minds, so it was acceptable to use surgery to change bodies in the name of wholeness.

Father O'Reilly knew a seminarian who was heading off to study at the Vatican. I boldly asked him to ask Pope Paul VI for a formal statement about gender confirmation surgery. The pope formed a committee to look into the matter, and the conclusion was that it is right to help people become whole by matching their physical reality to their psychological reality via surgery if the procedure is medically indicated. I was delighted to learn what the pope had to say; it mattered a great deal to me. I had already arrived at my personal moral sense of the matter, but the pope's weight in the world could help me convince others that gender confirmation surgery offered a chance to help people who were suffering terribly. It could also be a chance to shine as brightly as a Nobel

Prize–winner at Stanford, to become an expert in something new. Ambition and altruism were always linked in my psyche: I wanted to do good *and* be the best. For the most part, this compulsion has worked out well for patients and colleagues.

I hurled myself into the field of gender dysphoria at the same time that the project eventually called Interplast was expanding in Central America. Ninety-hour work weeks were the norm, but I was finding both avenues of work tremendously fulfilling. In the 1970s, I hosted the first international symposium on transsexualism and cofounded the Harry Benjamin International Gender Dysphoria Association, the first organization for physicians involved in gender confirmation surgery. It's now called the World Professional Association for Transgender Health (WPATH). I served as its second president and participated in developing the professional guidelines for treating gender dysphoria.

My experience with building better genitals came in surprisingly handy years later on a medical mission to Honduras, which in the early 1970s became the second country to welcome our teams. A seventeen-year-old boy came to the clinic in San Pedro Sula missing a penis. He'd contracted an infection at a house of ill repute and despite visits to several specialists who administered various antibiotics, the penis remained infected, swollen, and discolored. Eventually, it had turned black and fallen right off.

The team of volunteer Honduran surgeons and an American anesthesiologist who didn't know about my other work were sure this young fellow was beyond help.

"Don't worry," I said cheerfully. "We'll build him a new penis. I know how!" During the phalloplasty that followed, the assistant surgeon, Dr. Ortiz, called out to one of her colleagues, "Hey, Dr. Gonzalez! You should scrub in. This feels exactly like a real penis!"

SEVEN

INTERPLAST FLIES HIGH

Between 1968 and 1973, I made forty-five surgical visits to Mexicali with volunteer medical teams. Recruiting Stanford doctors and nurses was no problem. In fact, I was waylaid in the hallways of Stanford Hospital so many times by enthusiastic colleagues who wanted to talk about volunteering that I actually considered wearing a disguise to work. Individuals, corporations, and foundations stepped up to cover the modest budget of what we originally incorporated as the Mexico Medical Project. Stanford administered some funding, benefited from donor and community goodwill generated by our work, and conferred a boatload of cachet. The university and the Mexico Medical Project were working in concert, unofficially.

Most university officials cheered us on, although at the beginning, some expressed doubts that an international project would work. Others were simply surprised that I would want to go extramural. It was incipient Ass General disease: "We're Stanford! Why would you want to practice anywhere else?"

We also met with skepticism from some academics and members of county medical society ethics committees. Here are some of the criticisms-in-the-form-of-questions that I fielded, all no doubt well meant:

- Did we have buy-in from local physicians and their government, or were we imposing ourselves on the community?
- Were we making "parachute trips" — that is, dropping in, doing our thing, and leaving a mess behind?
- The American College of Surgeons (ACS) requires that a surgeon be on hand to treat post-op complications; how were we handling continuity of care?
- The ACS also forbids itinerant surgery at multiple sites; were we challenging that rule?
- Were we fostering dependency?
- Were we using people as guinea pigs?
- Was this medical imperialism — are we saying we're superior to local physicians?
- How can we keep things sterile in that dirty, dusty place? (I found the juxtaposition of those last two questions to be rather revealing.)

- How did we deal with cultural differences?

Luckily, we had an airtight answer for each of these challenges: Yes, we had the approval and participation of local medical societies and the permission of Mexican government at the state and federal level. Rotary Clubs on both sides of the border supported us financially and provided volunteer help. We also formed an alliance with the speech therapy department of the Autonomous University of Baja California, a state school whose main campus is in Mexicali. Granted, we weren't able to develop a bond with the surgery department there — because there wasn't one. Later, as we expanded, we worked closely with in-country medical schools all over the globe. We never practiced in places that didn't want us. And as it turned out, every place that initially turned down our offer of help or dismissed us eventually welcomed us. We were even invited back to Culiacán in 1970.

Continuity of care and sustainability were basic tenets of our project. Not only was postoperative supervision provided by expert local surgeons, but in Mexicali and, later, at each trip site, we also left behind an American physician assistant who stayed on for two weeks. Furthermore, we walked our talk: patients and physicians in the host country saw that we'd be back soon. The ACS rules had to do with retail surgery; they offered no guidelines for humanitarian service. Our method was respectful collaboration; our aim was to provide advanced training unavailable in low-resource countries. Patients weren't guinea pigs; we performed no experimental procedures.

As in any teaching hospital in America, they received sophisticated and meticulous surgical care observed by medical personnel eager to learn new techniques.

Regarding dust and dirt: I saw only great respect for the sterile field. If under-resourced hospitals didn't meet American standards of squeaky cleanliness, it wasn't because of lack of will but rather lack of resources. We supplied those resources, along with information about best practices. We were often humbled by how extraordinarily well our colleagues performed with minimal resources. They taught us to think about the ways that abundance can lead to wastefulness.

In Mexico and Central and South America, our teams always included at least one member who was fluent in Spanish, and we employed local translators. I set out to learn Spanish, reaching a level of expertise somewhere between not-so-caliente and ay-yi-yi — but I made myself understood, and my efforts were always welcomed effusively: "Doctor, you speak our language! *Gracias!*" We also learned cultural subtleties. For example, that it's never a waste of time to precede the examination of a patient with some gentle openers: "*¿Cómo le va? ¿Cómo ha amanecido? ¿Cómo esta su familia?*" (How is it going? How did you feel when you woke up? How is your family?) We dispensed more hugs than we did up north.

One set of wink-wink-nudge-nudge remarks we heard for years, and not just from critics but from colleagues who'd never participated: "You're just traveling to warm places so you can lay back, drink, dance, and fool around." The laid-back part was easily refuted by a look at our schedule sheets. We worked many more hours than at home, squeezing in more and more surgeries without sacrificing quality of care. (No volunteer doctor or nurse ever complained; in fact, it was quite the opposite. Time and again, they would exclaim some variation of "This is why I became a doctor!" or, "I want to do this for the rest of my life.") As for the drinking and dancing, yes, sure. And I'd add eating. Our great release after a fifteen-hour day of nonstop surgery was often crowding into the home of Phil and Luz for a fantastic meal and a few rounds of *cazuelas voladoras*, which translates loosely to "flying bowls," a delicious local cocktail built from tequila and citrus fruits and served in a clay vessel. Usually, Luz and Phil invited a mariachi band. There were no hammocks on the beach during our grueling trips, though; the team rarely left the hospital or clinic. The fooling around? All I can tell you is the rigors and joys of one of these trips create a kind of emotional crucible. Almost all our volunteer doctors and nurses, from medical students to seasoned practitioners, report that from their first international medical mission they became addicted to the peak experiences, psychic income, and camaraderie of these missions, a closeness that, over the years, led to lasting international friendships — and also to marriages and divorces.

Lars Vistnes, a plastic and reconstructive surgeon born and raised in Norway and educated in Canada and the U.S., joined the Stanford medical faculty in 1971. He was terrifically interested in the work we were doing in Mexicali as the first group to bring advanced reconstructive surgery to children and adults in developing countries who otherwise had no access to care. In his polite way, he pointed out that I knew nothing about finances and asked if he might take over that aspect of the project. In 1971, he turned the Mexico Medical Project into an official 501(c)(3) nonprofit, which meant donations were tax deductible. For every $10 donated, we provided $100 in free services. Lars, who died in 2016, succeeded me as chief of plastic surgery at Stanford. He made many Interplast trips to Guatemala, Honduras, Peru, and Samoa, where he worked in an open-air operating room. His specialty was oculoplastic surgery, and he was especially known for a novel procedure he devised to help Vietnam War vets — a way to reconstruct orbital bones and eyelids so soldiers who had lost an eye could be fitted with a good-looking prosthetic instead of a patch or an awkward fake. When I consider Lars's work, I think about how medical advances that seem inevitable and commonplace today, such as microsurgery, the transplantation of organs and digits, or the placement of aesthetically pleasing prosthetic eyes, required a passionate visionary pushing the boundaries of received wisdom.

By 1970, I had begun laying the groundwork for expansion into Central American countries and beyond. So, the name Mexico Medical Project felt outdated. I put out the word that we were looking for a handle that was sexy and conveyed our mission — delivering free plastic and reconstructive surgery all over the developing world to impoverished people who otherwise had no options. A Stanford anesthesiologist from Wales, Vernon Thomas, wrote to a professor of his in England for suggestions. One day Vernon called me and shouted, "I have it! I have it! *Interplast*, for *inter*national *plast*ic surgery." We registered it right away. That name stuck until 2010, when the organization became ReSurge International, for *recon*structive *surge*ry. Also, in English, to resurge means *to rise again*, and in Spanish *to reappear* — both apt descriptions of what patients experience when their damaged bodies are repaired.

Letters went out to government officials all over Central America, to medical professors, hospital heads, and the chief medical officers of the U.S. Agency for International Development (USAID), offering surgery, instruction by Stanford professors, and free equipment and supplies. I also wrote formal letters to First Ladies, all of whom supported projects involving services for children. My aim was to set up personal visits, the best way to get things done. The first positive response came from Honduras, and I immediately arranged to get together with the minister of education and the minister of foreign affairs. Kees and Phil joined me in Tegucigalpa for the meeting, which took place at 8 a.m. on a Sunday morning. The rather sleepy ministers thanked us but told us they already had help in the capital; an American plastic surgeon from Miami had come and corrected four cases of hypospadias — a birth defect in boys where the opening of the urethra is in the wrong spot. But they liked my plan, which combined education and healthcare and would burnish their reputations. They decided that the coastal city of San Pedro Sula, to the north, could use our services. "I'll call a doctor there who knows about these needs," one of the ministers said. He picked up the phone and spoke to Dr. René Bendaña, a ninety-two-year-old urologist. "Hello, René," he said, "I have three visiting experts here who would like to evaluate our needs for unrepaired cleft lips, hypospadias, and burn scar contractures. I'll send them up there. They will arrive at 11:45 a.m." We were driven to the airport, and we took a cab to Hospital Leonardo Martinez V, a 110-year-old public hospital where many of the physicians of San Pedro Sula spent their mornings tending to the needs of the poor. We were quickly told that Dr. Bendaña had gone home. At his home, we were told he had gone to his farm. We retreated to the bar of the Gran Sula Hotel to discuss next steps over *cervezas.*

Providence arranged for a friendly, dynamic local physician to overhear our conversation. A doer of good himself, he liked what he heard and addressed us in excellent English. "I am Dr. Luis Bueso, a pediatrician. I have experience with a group of gringos coming here to help with surgery and ending up being kicked out by the Colegio Médico. They were my good friends, the Americans, and highly qualified, but they had some degree of naïveté. They charged patients who could afford it on a sliding scale and donated back to the hospital to help the poor obtain free medical care. The Colegio thought that perhaps this was another instance of the gringos coming here and making money at the expense of the Honduran economy. And out they went.

"But if you follow my advice, I will protect you, and

you will be okayed by the Colegio Médico when they send out their evaluators to check you out. In my practice, I have many, many cleft lip and palates for you, many hand injuries, many congenital hand anomalies."

Luis instantly felt like a brother. After a half hour's talk, we decided that Dr. Bueso would prepare the way by explaining our collaborative model to his colleagues. I would return with a team for a needs-assessment visit, at which time Interplast and the local Colegio would, I hoped, sign a formal letter of agreement to launch an international surgery program.

It all worked beautifully, and it continues to do so. San Pedro Sula's population has more than doubled, to half a million, and patients come from all over the country to be treated by teams from Interplast/ReSurge led by talented Honduran doctors.

One of the first cases Interplast handled in Honduras demonstrates nicely the efficacy and synergy of our system. Javier made his living with a machete, cutting banana bunches — some weighing more than fifty pounds — from the tree, often with one stroke. He worked hard and liked to relax with Salva Vida, the 10 percent beer introduced to local agricultural workers as an alternative to high-octane Flor de Caña — a strong rum, the over-indulgence in which was said to play a part in the many grisly and sometimes fatal machete injuries in Honduras — a phenomenon known locally as Collins syndrome, after Collins & Co., the British firm that manufactured the machetes. Javier came to Interplast suffering from a serious but nonlethal case of Collins syndrome resulting from a love-triangle machete fight. He'd lost a cheek and part of his mouth.

Javier's case proved to be a wonderful teaching opportunity. The required treatment involved sophisticated techniques that weren't generally known in Honduras at the time. Three Honduran surgeons teamed with three American surgeons to perform a complicated repair job while local surgeons, residents, and medical students observed. We carried a huge skin flap on a living pedicle from the chest to the surface of the cheek and transferred skin and tissue from the forehead to the inside lining of the cheek. Two skin grafts were taken from Javier's leg to replace the tissue taken from the chest and forehead. The flaps were in place for a full three weeks. These procedures were accomplished without a complication. I can't say how the love affair turned out, but the surgery was a success; Javier looked fine, and he went back to work. Not only that, but the Honduran medical community, their skills expanded and confidence boosted, understood they were capable of complicated surgery even in a low-resource area.

During Interplast's first five years, we provided surgery for 750 patients in Mexico, Honduras, Guatemala, Nicaragua, and Samoa on an annual budget of less than $18,000 a year. Getting our volunteer doctors and nurses (and usually a social worker who served as trip secretary) to surgical sites was an interesting process. That old Dodge van of mine, with air horns mounted on the roof and two extra gas tanks installed below, was a cheap ride to Mexicali, but it was slow and impractical once we expanded to other countries. For a while, we used the pro bono services kindly offered by the physician-pilots of the Flying Doctors organization. That was fine for personnel, but their light planes couldn't handle our cargo, sometimes as many as forty heavy boxes of supplies and equipment. One time, I'd commissioned 350 clay bowls to go down with the supplies so Interplast teams could have parties in Honduras with the right equipment for *cazuelas voladoras*. In order to make altitude over the mountains in a small Cessna, the trip leader had to jettison the bowls.

The answer was the Interplast Airforce. With the help of two retired pilots, Bob Bell and George Chippendale, we purchased a sturdy used DC-3 — safe, stable, and capable of carrying great weight. Teams were able to be at work mere hours after takeoff from Northern California.

Unlike the ill-fated Interplast Navy, the Interplast Airforce worked well. Until it didn't. After a couple of years of too many unscheduled landings for cylinder replacements, we were forced to find other transportation solutions. I considered asking the real military for help with transportation. Back in 1962, during the Cuban Missile Crisis, young physicians were worried about being drafted. Like many of my Yale colleagues, I'd joined the Army Reserves to avoid the possibility of active service. That meant a reserve meeting every other week in downtown New Haven and a few weeks a year of service at an army hospital. Early in my reserve career, I was flying to reserve summer service at the burn unit of the San Antonio Military Medical Center, and I realized that my seatmate was the legendary plastic surgeon

Truman G. Blocker, who became the president of the University of Texas. His words of wisdom to me were "Boy, you've got your insignia upside down!" When I moved to California, the meetings were at the Presidio of San Francisco. I rose to become a captain in the reserves, and I was interested in moving up the ranks because as a major I could add a line item to the budget: a community-oriented international health program, with young reservists as volunteers. Interplast could use the money for transportation. I had all the plans in place, ready to submit, but I didn't get the promotion . . . because I'd once gone AWOL. I was at Madigan Army Medical Center in Tacoma, Washington, when Judy was about to give birth by Caesarian to our fifth and youngest child, Louise, and I flew down to Stanford Hospital to be with her. When I put in for a promotion to major, a supervising physician who knew about the AWOL episode said, "I can't recommend Laub; he's too slippery." I stayed on for a bit after not making major, but my reserve days were over — and, in my view, another fine plan had been dashed because of ridiculous rules upheld by people who couldn't see the bigger picture.

After the grounding of the Interplast Airforce, we turned to commercial airlines, which we still use today. Doctors pay for their own transportation and the organization takes care of nurses and residents. Social worker Amy Laden became a vital part of the team in the mid-70s, finding foster homes for patients, doctors, and nurses visiting Stanford, organizing surgical trips, and using her brilliant interpersonel skills to keep everyone on an even keel. Today, she's the director of international services at ReSurge.

My wife, Judy, played a crucial role in the early days of Interplast, hosting visiting doctors, nurses, and patients in our home. After my first trip to Culiacán in 1967, for example, two of the Mexican nurses came to visit for several weeks. We turned the garage into a make-shift bedroom so the visitors could have ours. Then we moved to a bigger house, and it was filled to capacity when Louise was born in August 1969. Phil brought up six children from Mexicali who needed difficult surgery, and they stayed with us until foster homes could be found for them. Judy somehow managed a new baby, our four other children, and six extras.

When our youngest was travel-worthy, we'd some-times pile all the kids in the Dodge van and the whole family would accompany me to Mexicali. While I did surgery, Judy and the kids helped out at a Catholic mission. My older son, Don Jr., known as D2, says these trips made a big impression on him and played a role in his decision to become a plastic surgeon. He's participated in more than a dozen missions to five different countries, including Vietnam.

In a later batch of kids from Mexicali at our house, one eleven-year-old boy, Jose Luis, bonded with D2, who was the same age. Jose Luis was determined to stay with us; he cuddled up to me and called me Papa. He'd been burned while jumping through a tire that had burning rags in it. He was a great kid but a challenge for Judy. His right arm was contracted to his side and needed to be released. Judy took him to San Mateo County Hospital for surgery. Afterward, he was put into an airplane splint, which holds the arm away from the body at a ninety-degree angle. When Judy brought Jose Luis home, she drove into the garage. The phone was ringing, so she ran to answer it, and when she hurried back to the car, Jose Luis was riding D2's bike down the street, airplane splint and all, his hospital gown flapping wide open in the back. Judy had a tough time controlling him. D2 helped, even emptying bedpans and sharing his things. After Jose Luis healed, he focused more on playing with and teasing the girls. We took him camping with us in the Wind River Mountains of Idaho. Judy had a soft spot for this lively, fun-loving boy. She was also attached to Maria, a sweet, shy woman in her thirties with a large tumor on her spinal column who stayed with us. And she was amused by Pancho Villa Velasquez, a forty-eight-year-old man who recuperated at our house after surgery. He was with us during Halloween, and all of the trick-or-treaters went down the hallway to Pancho's bedroom so he could see their costumes and give them candy.

There was five-year-old Ana, whose eye had been torn out by a springing wire while her father was fixing something. She stayed with us while she was waiting for a false eye. A quiet girl, Ana was fond of our daughters. Judy took the kids to the pool and asked Ana in Spanish if she could swim. She said, "*Si*," walked down the stairs into the water, and never came up. Judy had to jump in and pull her out.

What Judy calls her most interesting challenge came

right after the first group of children arrived at our house. All the children, ours included, had to be treated for head lice. Judy called the local pediatrician. He said he'd never seen head lice and begged her to bring in the kids so he could take a look. The treatment then was several applications of Kwell shampoo and laundering everything in sight. Interplast introduced new hope in the lives of impoverished children. I'm afraid Interplast also introduced head lice to the Palo Alto Unified School District. Judy, as always, took it in stride.

An overheard conversation in a bar had launched our work in Honduras. Three years later, the same method got Interplast into Africa. In 1973, Dave Dibbell, in Houston for a plastic surgery meeting, was having a drink in the bar of the Ambassador Hotel very late one night. He couldn't help but hear a loud declaration from a group at the next table. "Bringing good bull semen to Africa is the world's best project." The speaker was the president of a foundation dedicated to improving cattle breeding in the U.S. and developing nations by supplying bull semen from superior livestock for artificial insemination. Dave leaned over and chimed right in. "No . . . it's not semen that's the most important thing," he said. "The most important thing is correcting the disparity in distribution of medical services between countries." Then he called me from a pay phone, waking me up. "Hello, Don. I'm here at a bar in Houston telling this guy that Interplast surgery is much better than improving the cattle in Africa with semen from American bulls. Tell him how great our project is and why he should support it." I did just that, then surprised the hell out of the guy by saying, "I'm in California, but I can meet you for lunch tomorrow in Houston to discuss details." I didn't mention that I was already scheduled to take an early morning flight to Houston to attend the same meeting as Dr. Dibbell.

That lunch resulted in the foundation's funding a needs-assessment trip and our first surgical mission to Lesotho, the small, landlocked nation entirely surrounded by South Africa. Thus was launched a long and successful collaboration among Interplast volunteers, surgeons in Lesotho, and enthusiastic faculty at the University of Cape Town. Hundreds of patients have benefited, and scores of surgical residents have honed their skills and opened their hearts to the joys of psychic income.

EIGHT

SHAPE SHIFTING

When I first became involved in gender confirmation surgery, "passability" was one of the key ways to gauge whether the transition from male to female was successful. Learning stereotypical female behavior was considered important to adjustment. By the 1980s, the Gender Dysphoria Program's ideas had evolved as we came to understand that passing undetectably as another sex isn't important to everyone. There's no right way to be a post-operative trans person, nor is the word "postoperative" always appropriate — some transgender and gender-fluid people want breast augmentation or removal and some don't; some want genital surgery and some don't.

But back in the late 1960s and early 1970s, in the early days of the program, medical professionals dealing with trans people focused on surgery and established an international organization — the Harry Benjamin International Gender Dysphoria Association — and developed a set of guidelines for the safe, successful, and humane surgical treatment of gender dysphoria.

Surgery was the culmination of a lengthy and complex process, each step of which was documented by an attorney, from the sharing of expectations to the disclosure of risks to informed consent for the procedure. Before surgery, the patient would spend a year or two on hormones appropriate to the new sex and undergo whatever cosmetic procedures would allow them to pass undetectably. At the beginning, all of our patients were undergoing a male-to-female shift, so our emphasis was on living as a female, adjusting psychologically to the new sex, earning a living, and having a fulfilling social, romantic, and sexual life.

One of the dumbest things I ever did was to invite Truman Capote to teach trans women feminine behavior. It didn't seem so crazy at the time; he thought it was intriguing and eventually signed on to narrate a documentary on transsexualism, *Second Chance*, that seems never to have gotten made. But he didn't have much advice to impart about passing; his thing was stylized effeminate behavior. After that, we started what I called the Finishing School, a series of workshops led by cis women — women whose gender identity matches their sex assigned at birth — designed to teach trans women who were to be our patients "socially acceptable feminine graces" such as how to sit or how to bend over to pick things up. The patients seemed to appreciate it. Eventually, the Finishing School was obsolete.

There was some rancor — patients balked at the lengthy run-up to surgery. They would say things like, "We want surgery and you ivory-tower gatekeepers are delaying our right to surgery by making artificial rules." Gradually, some came around to the rules. At the same time, our patients educated us about what really makes a happy change of gender. Eventually, passing became passé.

Many of my transgender patients have become friends, and they enjoy teasing me about the raising of my consciousness over the years. Sandy Stone, now a professor emeritus at the University of Texas and founder of the academic field of transgender studies, likes to tell stories about the times we clashed during preparations for her gender confirmation surgery in 1977. "I owe Dr. Laub a lifelong debt of gratitude," she recently told a radio host. "He's a good surgeon. But he's a tough gatekeeper." The first time Sandy walked into my office wearing jeans, work boots, and a long beard, she said, in a rather macho voice, "I'm interested in a sex change." I said, "To what?'"

Sandy entered the program, which required two years of taking hormones, undergoing extensive electrolysis to remove facial and body hair, and living as the desired sex. Sandy remembered one of our meetings during her transition when the beard and the macho voice were long gone. "I sit down, and Don says, 'Why aren't you dressed like a woman?' I'm wearing jeans and a T-shirt. I say, 'I *am* dressed like a woman.' Don says, 'No, you're not.' I say, 'Have you looked out the window recently?'

"When I was about to have the vaginoplasty, Don asked me if I was 100 percent sure about going ahead with it. I said I was 99.9 percent sure and that anyone who was 100 percent sure about anything was probably crazy. I mean, we all have doubts. I said, 'I'm an adult. I can take responsibility for my actions. This is informed consent. If I made a mistake, it's my fault, not yours. Let's go.' Don frowned and said, 'I'm sorry. You're not eligible. If you're not 100 percent sure, I can't do the surgery. It's canceled.'"

Sandy was shocked. Luckily, Judy Van Maasdam, the wonderful social worker who was the coordinator of the Gender Dysphoria Program, intervened and convinced me to accept, grudgingly that 99.9 percent was a pretty darned good percentage in the real world, as opposed to Laub World. Van Maasdam would go on to become one of the most highly regarded behavioral scientists in the field of gender dysphoria and a member of the board of the World Professional Association for Transgender Health. Three months later, Judy called Sandy in for a rescripted meeting. Sandy remembers, "Each of us needs a particular thing. I wanted surgery, and I didn't want to be thought of as crazy. Don didn't want to have to let go of control. So, we met and Don said, 'Are you ready for surgery?' And I said, 'Yes!'"

Another requirement that was dropped, one that seems painfully antiquated now, was that the patients were only accepted into the Gender Dysphoria Program if they intended to be heterosexual after the surgery. The outrage of the transgender community helped enlighten us on that issue. Though the relationship between the community and the program was warm and close, it could be contentious; we were still gatekeepers, making the ultimate decision about whom we deemed eligible for surgery.

I knew intuitively that the surgical work we were doing was vital and valuable and far more effective than behavioral modification in easing the discomfort of patients with gender dysphoria. But there'd been no credible, evidence-based academic study of the efficacy of surgical rehabilitation for gender dysphoria — we had no solid statistics to convince the skeptics. A crisis led to me undertaking the first such study.

From the beginning, gender confirmation surgery felt like a form of helping people that was absolutely right. It gave me the same feeling that I'd gotten on Interplast trips: *This is what I'm for. This is my purpose. This is why I became a doctor.* Not everyone agreed with me.

In 1971, my boss and mentor Robert Chase called to tell me that the president of the university wanted me to stop doing gender confirmation surgery at Stanford. A donor from conservative Orange County was threatening to withhold a gift of $2 million. I was so upset that I found out where the president parked his car, waited for him, and introduced myself. "Sir," I said civilly, "I think you're making a mistake." He said, with equal civility, "It's not a mistake. It's two million dollars." I said, "You don't understand." He said, "*You* don't understand," and drove off. I actually cried.

I thought about it all night and came up with a plan. I presented the work of the Gender Dysphoria Program at surgery grand rounds, the formal meeting at which interesting cases are presented to senior colleagues and residents. I stacked the audience with distinguished physicians who would serve, in essence, as a jury and asked them a key question: Is gender confirmation surgery a bona fide academic pursuit? The men and women of the brain trust answered yes. Surely this would impress the president.

I also tried to made him happy with a technicality: the actual gender confirmation surgery would be done by me and other members of the Stanford clinical faculty *not* at Stanford Hospital but at San Mateo County's public hospital, then called the Harold D. Chope Community Hospital and now the San Mateo Medical Center. Nothing visible changed — the Gender Dysphoria Program remained at Stanford, but the president could say honestly to the disgruntled donor that Stanford didn't do the surgery.

I went on to do the first formal academic study of gender confirmation surgery, interviewing and/or treating 2,000 patients to determine whether changing the body of the gender dysphoric person to fit the mind rather than vice versa substantially helped the patient. The answer: it did, in at least 75 percent of patients surveyed. More recent investigations, such as a 2007 study done in England by researchers at the University Hospitals of Leicester, show even higher numbers.

I had faced down a biased donor and saved the Gender Dysphoria Program at Stanford. But later that same year, an iconoclastic nun forced me to face some biases of my own.

NINE

THE PRESIDENT VERSUS THE NUN

Sister Jane, the surgeon-nun, was furious with me. "You are betraying the poor!" she shouted. That's certainly not what I'd meant to do when I led an Interplast team to the remote Maryknoll mission hospital in the western highlands of Guatemala. And that's not at all how I saw the decision that so disturbed Sister Jane. But getting roundly rebuked by a righteously raging nun can shake the worldview of a man who, as the product of a Jesuit education, thought he was doing a pretty good job of consecrating his life to helping others and doing the right thing.

Back in 1970, Guatemala had become the third site for Interplast surgeries, after Mexico and Honduras. The nation's minister of health and the U.S. Agency for International Development (USAID) welcomed the project. Most important, we had the enthusiastic support of the country's first lady, Alida España, wife of President Carlos Arana Osorio. She decided how revenue from the national lottery would be used, and she wanted to help children. We promised to provide her with a good project to match her good intentions.

One of our first destinations was the hard-to-reach town of Jacaltenango in a mile-high valley ringed by the Cuchumatan Mountains, not far from the Mexican border. The Maryknoll convent and hospital there, headed by Sister Jane, served subsistence farm families who were members of the indigenous Jakaltek Mayan community.

I'd realized immediately that Sister Jane was nothing like the nuns I'd known growing up in Milwaukee, though that was her hometown, too. The first time I met her, when I made a preliminary needs-assessment trip to the hospital, she'd pointed to an urn in a niche above the stone hearth of the convent's dining hall. "Those," she said, "are the ashes of the Rules of the Maryknoll Order." And when our first team of three surgeons and an anesthesiologist arrived in Jacaltenango in 1971, Sister Jane was showing a film about birth control methods — from condoms to pills with no mention of the rhythm method — on the wall of a sixteenth-century church. A large gathering of local folk watched with intense interest.

Getting to Jacaltenango had required an eight-hour drive on a one-lane unpaved road that had been completed just one month before we arrived. When I'd visited six months earlier to line up cases, I'd had to make most of the journey by mule, on precarious cliffside trails. The new road, all curves and switchbacks, was really just one step up from a trail, too narrow for safe driving. A swerve to the right or left could mean a thousand-foot plunge.

I was driving a blue two-wheel-drive pickup truck loaded with four 2,000-gallon tanks of nitrous oxide — laughing gas — lying side by side in the truck bed. We'd stuffed soft supplies between the tanks to immobilize them, but the rough road caused nerve-wracking bouncing nonetheless. We pictured the tanks tilting the truck right off a cliff. Richard Siegel was riding shotgun in the truck. A third-year plastic surgery resident at Stanford, he was capable and enthusiastic. "Rick," I said, "stick your head out the window and tell me about my relationship with the road. I can't see anything but sky!"

"A little to the left," he called. "There's a curve ahead." Then, "Back up around the switchback until your rear wheel goes off the road, otherwise you'll never make the turn." Surgeon Howard Holderness and anesthesiologist Vern Thomas were behind us in a jeep. The drive was harrowing but beautiful — hillsides impossibly terraced with fields of corn, potatoes, and barley, neatly planted and precisely preened; in the distance, steep green mountains were draped in fog.

The thirteen Maryknollers, all in civilian dress, three of them physicians, were good company — highly educated, caring, well prepared, pragmatic, energetic, and cocky. The nuns were justifiably proud of their hospital, established in 1958; every piece of equipment had been brought in on mule-back. They were fiercely devoted to the indigenous Mayan people of Guatemala, who were, Sister Jane told us, kept impoverished, landless, and voiceless by the privileged ruling class, descendants of Europeans who owned huge farms and factories. The Maryknoll nuns were living examples of liberation theology, an interpretation of Christian scriptures emphasizing a special duty to free the poor from oppression. The sisters supported a political agenda of change — through legislation, if possible; if not, then through revolution.

Especially strong in Latin America, liberation theology was first espoused in the 1950s, and by the early 1970s, it was in full flower. The Vatican and the U.S. government were made uncomfortable by liberation theology; the emphasis on uplifting the oppressed and redressing income inequality had, to those institutions, an unpleasant whiff of Marxism. Sister Jane and like-minded nuns and priests working in Latin America were courageously committed to social justice. Later, I would learn that this stance put them at great personal risk. Many of our friends in Guatemala were killed by government-sanctioned death squads, including Father Stanley Rother, a priest from Oklahoma who was murdered for his work with the poor in Santiago Atitlán. He was recently beatified.

Surgery on our lineup of patients began early on the morning after our arrival, in a pleasant operating room with a big window overlooking the town soccer field, nearby green foothills, and, in the far distance, the mountains of Chiapas, Mexico, forty miles away. Jacaltenango wasn't electrified, but the hospital had a generator. There were no telephones; the nuns communicated with church headquarters in the capital by short-wave radio every morning at 8 a.m.

Sister Jane scrubbed in to observe the first surgery of the day, repairing the cleft lip of a Jakaltek boy. Some of the operating room nurses were nuns and others were local women. Not long after we began, the mission's radio technician entered the OR and quietly informed us that the president of Guatemala had just radioed to say he was sending his personal helicopter to pick me up. El Presidente's good friend, the industrialist and hotelier Jorge Kong, had been shot in the jaw during an assassination attempt. The helicopter would arrive shortly.

"You're not going, of course," Sister Jane declared flatly. "You have these children to care for." I told her that since Interplast was allowed to work in Guatemala at the pleasure of the president, I felt I had to accede to his request for the sake of future good deeds. Sister Jane declared that I was letting her down. I declared that I wasn't. When we finished the surgery, Sister Jane and I stepped out of the OR to finish our argument. Rick Siegel told me afterward that the team, preparing the next patient, could hear escalating mutual invective and a few thumps that sounded like someone pounding a table or kicking a wall.

I told Sister Jane that Rick would come with me and that while we were gone Howard and Vern would keep working; we'd be back soon. A patient needed me in the capital, I said, and my helping him wouldn't hurt my patients here. Furthermore, I thought to myself, this little detour would help solidify my relationship with the ruling class and thus secure Interplast's place in Guatemala. I was, I told Sister Jane, outside of politics in the conventional sense of left versus right, or communism versus capitalism. Sister Jane countered that no one was outside politics. Things got heated, and that's when Sister Jane declared vehemently that I was betraying the poor. I noted emphatically that she was missing the big picture. She replied, even more emphatically, that I was the one missing the big picture. In Guatemala, she said, 2 percent of the population owned 72 percent of the land, a great deal of it stolen from indigenous farmers. Though President Arana was admired by many for providing the Mayan people with schools, wells, and clinics, he was also a military strongman whose repressive government detained and disappeared political opponents, student leaders, workers active in trade unions, and anyone thought to support indigenous guerrillas seeking to topple the regime rigged against them. That political order had come to power in 1954 when the American CIA toppled democratically elected, progressive president Jacobo Árbenz. At the height of the Red Scare, anticommunist members of Eisenhower's cabinet, who also had ties to the American-owned United Fruit Company, a major player in Guatemala, convinced Ike that Árbenz must have communist leanings. The strongest evidence was that he'd initiated a plan to return to indigenous people land taken from them by the United Fruit Company. Today, Sister Jane said, many of the people disappearing on Arana's watch were victims of state-sponsored death squads, and right-wing activist Jorge Kong, the patient

I'd been tapped to treat in the capital, was implicated in these extrajudicial murders. This was news to me and deeply unsettling — but I still felt it was right to help a patient in real need for the greater good.

The beauty of Interplast, I told Sister Jane, is that we're able to enter into the midst of conflict and controversy and make friends with each faction. Our concern was to alleviate the obvious unequal distribution of medical care — the discrepancy between those with access and those without, the haves and the have-nots. This was amazingly similar to the goals of socialism, so we were the friends of the left, who could see that we were taking care of the people. We were friends of American-trained Guatemalan physicians who represented conservatism and helped legitimize our work in the country; we were friends of the executive branch of the U.S. through the chief in-country medical officer of the U.S. Agency for International Development, who made a tour with us of every hospital in the countries that wanted our help; and we were friends of the Guatemalan government, who provided us with recognition and helicopter transportation. We were friends of the poor because we repaired deformities for free, which helped them immensely. We weren't betraying the poor. Sister Jane still thought I shouldn't go to the capital, but we agreed to disagree.

We returned to the OR, and our team began reconstructing the partially paralyzed face of a four-year-old boy using grafts of fascia from his thigh to connect working muscles of mastication to other parts of his mouth and to his eye to remobilize these areas. We were halfway through the surgery when we saw through the OR window a new yellow and white Sikorsky helicopter landing on the soccer field. Within minutes, hundreds of local residents had flocked to witness this unprecedented sight. I instructed Howard and Vern to finish the case, which was going smoothly. To Sister Jane's obvious disgust, Rick and I, each with a bag of surgical instruments, ran out to the helicopter. The pilot insisted that we couldn't make it back up and over the 10,000-foot pass carrying the extra weight of an assistant. I persuaded him that Rick was the skinniest man on our team and wouldn't make a difference.

We made it over the pass, then flew low over the glorious countryside. The president's pilot asked in Spanish, first anxiously and then angrily, if we'd seen his map case. I discovered I was sitting on it. He unzipped the case and removed not a map but a long, shiny German Luger. He took off the safety and cocked it. Rick and I feared momentarily that the emergency house call was a ruse and we were about to be terminated for consorting with commie nuns. Perhaps because of the looks on our faces, the pilot hastily explained, "It's only to return the fire of the guerillas in the jungle if they shoot up at us."

The trip that took eight hours by pickup truck was surprisingly short in a chopper. At the Guatemala City airport, we were met by Kong's crew, tough men with scars and automatic weapons, who ushered us into a Mercedes-Benz 600 and followed in an armada of VW buses. One of our handlers let us know right away that Jorge Kong had been treated by a local oral surgeon and

that he was in good shape. Our job would be to exam-
ine the patient, check out the work of the Guatemalan
doctor, determine whether Kong needed further surgery,
and provide a plan for future care.

I asked the handler how Kong had been shot. "He was
riding in his Chrysler with his bodyguards," the fellow
replied, "followed by a VW bus full of more bodyguards.
The car stopped at a traffic light behind a pickup truck. A
.50 caliber machine gun quickly came up from the back
of the truck and started firing — *pop pop pop pop*. The
driver was killed; the bodyguard took cover to protect
himself. Jorge got out on the right side, ducked below the
open door, and got off about six rounds at the assassin."

"Where's Jorge's car now?" I asked.

"In a warehouse."

I saw an opportunity, and knowing that our patient
was in no danger, I took it. "We'll need to photograph the
car," I said. "Dr. Siegel and I are studying ballistics and
bullet wounds. We've made a film about damage to the
body related to muzzle velocity." Our handler got on the
two-way radio, and we made a U-turn.

Kong's car was a Chrysler 300, the biggest model,
with bullet holes sprayed across the windshield. The bul-
lets indeed appeared to have been .50 caliber and very low
velocity. We studied the damage to the vehicle, tried to
reenact the whole scene, photographed all aspects, and
made notes.

Then it was on to the Kong compound, a fortress-
mansion behind a six-foot wall topped with shards of glass
and strands of barbed wire. At each corner of the wall, a

guard with a submachine gun sat on a little basket-like platform. Inside, we were ushered past plenty of glistening marble and thick Persian carpets to Kong's bedroom. The patient, dressed in burgundy silk pajamas and robe, lay glowering in a four-poster bed elevated two steps above the floor. Three associates stood at his bedside. He dismissed them. "*¿Que pasó, Jorge?*" I asked pleasantly.

"Gohdahm cohmminists!" he said, hampered by his bandaged jaw. That was his answer to nearly every question we asked about the incident.

The bullet had entered at the angle of the jaw, skittered along the mandible beneath the soft tissue, and exited through the chin without breaking any bones. We removed the dressing and examined him closely. He had no facial nerve injury and his jaw was stabilized nicely by the dental arch bar splints placed by the Guatemalan doctor. He wasn't likely to need reconstructive surgery. We outlined his follow-up care and assured him that the first doctor had done an excellent job. He assured us that he had no affection for "gohdahm cohmminists."

Jorge Kong opened a drawer in his nightstand, took out his checkbook and a pen, and began writing as he asked, "What is your fee?" I answered, "Nothing now, but do us a big favor, a political favor when the time comes for one. We want to work in this country, and there will be those who want us out of here. Help us at that moment." Jorge smiled, rang a bell for a servant, and instructed the man to fetch his two sons immediately. The young men, in their late twenties, arrived in a heartbeat. Jorge told them to remember me, Dr. Laub, and never forget that

I'd come to Jorge's aid that day. Anytime in their lives, he said, if Dr. Laub needed assistance of any kind, even long after he, Jorge, was gone, they were to provide whatever was asked. They studied me and Rick for a moment, then nodded obediently. Much later, Rick told me, "I saw his checkbook; he had written $10,000 U.S. on the check, and I admired you very much for turning it down. But I never really understood why you didn't take the money!" I declined because I felt that possible future protection was priceless. And given the way the government warmed to Interplast, I feel that Jorge did intervene on our behalf.

But maybe I should have accepted the check.

Jorge's sons took Rick and me to a restaurant for a lunch of fine porterhouse steaks. We sat with our backs to the wall, flanked by armed guards. Perhaps a bit impishly, I asked the Kong brothers what they thought should be done to help the poor. To my surprise, they said they favored increased taxes on the rich. The political beliefs of these young men were far different from their father's.

On the helicopter ride back to the Jacaltenango, Rick and I were giddy over our enormous adventure. We'd stepped into the world of those who ruled without rules and had returned unscathed; we'd seen a bullet-riddled Chrysler, gotten a pledge of eternal help from a powerful man, had a good steak, and left with a great story. I felt high. And when we arrived at the mission hospital . . . I was suddenly knocked back to earth. Sister Jane was well and truly pissed. She barely spoke to me the rest of the trip, except to make clear that she felt I had deserted a poor Jakaltek boy who needed my help in order to serve a rich and evil man. By her lights, I should have refused to go; that would have made a mighty statement. I had blown a chance to show that all people are equal. That radio message from the president, she thought, could have provided the chance for liberation theology to strike a mighty blow against a deadly regime. The oppressors wanted to land in the very heart of her territory to try to snatch a precious possession — me — away from the poor. She'd hoped to make a point by withholding that treasure, and she had been sure I'd help her fight the arrogant entitlement of the powerful. Instead, I cheerfully let myself be snatched. She was incensed.

And I was crestfallen. I had done the right thing according to Hippocrates: I had taken care of my patient without any regard for his social or economic status. At least one outcome of my decision was good: protection of Interplast. But at least one outcome of my decision was terrible. My medical priorities led to the thought, *How could I neglect a human with a machine gun wound in his face who was asking me for help?* Sister Jane's priorities led her to the thought, *How could you abandon the needy to help a nefarious oligarch?* We were miles apart in our views. That was painful to me, and the pain lingered.

Four years later, Sister Jane and I were both in Chicago to attend a meeting of the American College of Surgeons. I invited her to breakfast.

"Good morning, Sister," I greeted her. "Good to see you again."

"Hello, Don. What do you know?"

"I know that *Collegeum Pulsationum Durarum*, the

school of hard knocks, is a good teacher. I've been thinking a lot about that time when Interplast first came to
Jacaltenango."

We each presented our point of view once again.

"I think you could have shown the capitalists that you
had an equal obligation to those Jakaltek children," Sister
Jane said. "They have plenty of arrogance and they abuse
capitalism, but they respect the raw courage of the North
Americans. You could have taught them something."

"Shouldn't you help a person, rich or poor, if he's
shot?" I said.

"The Jakaltek needed an example of someone standing up to those bastards who take advantage of them;
they're economic slave masters."

"But Interplast must stay in a neutral political zone,
or we can't do our job."

"You let me down."

"I am friends, truly friends, with both the left and
right. The rich ones are people, too. Real friendship counts
for a lot, and it's powerful in decision-making."

"What you did showed poor judgment. It was wrong."

I tried again. "Bullshit." Not the best approach. "There's
a commonality in medicine that crosses every political
boundary, every '–ism.' As my wife, Judy, says, 'Every
patient stands equal in front of a doctor.' Poor is equal to
rich and the rich patient has rights equal to the poor one.
Interplast has no agenda except to help." Befriending the
ruling class, I said, was the tactic I used to gain permission
to treat those with no access to medical care. I still thought
that if I'd become a figurative martyr for the cause — been

a splinter in the rear end of the elitist "haves" and refused to treat Jorge Kong — we might not have had the political protection we needed to continue our work in Guatemala. And the Jakaltek boy with a paralyzed face had not, I believed, suffered from my absence.

Sister Jane smiled. "Perhaps by more skillfully managing your tactics, you could allow everyone concerned to rise to a higher level of understanding."

"That's my approach exactly, Sister. And I still think that we can heal the whole world with reconstructive surgery."

We understood each other's stance — but by the end of breakfast, we were still miles apart about that helicopter ride. I thought I was following Aristotle, who argued in his *Nicomachean Ethics* that "virtue makes the choice right." Sister Jane went further back, into ancient Greek history, and heeded Plato, who tells us in the *Republic* that justice and happiness are intertwined; those who choose justice have more ordered souls and live happier lives than those who don't.

For decades, the incident troubled me. When you know you're right, how can you be wrong? Ultimately, I realized two things. First, Sister Jane and I shared a basic premise — that all people are equal. Second, I could have taken an intermediate course by making radio contact with the capital to find out how Jorge Kong was doing. If his condition was stable, I could have made a small political statement and supported Sister Jane while still serving the president; I could have remained with the boy until the end of his operation, which would have taken less than an hour, and *then* gone to the bedside of Jorge Kong. It took me forty years to think of this compromise. This modicum of evolution wouldn't have been possible without Sister Jane's righteous rage, fueled by love, pushing me to a higher level of thinking.

TEN

THE GUN THAT WON THE WEST

By 1986, volunteer Interplast surgical teams had done more than 2,500 operations in Ecuador, at sites ranging from big hospitals in Quito, the capital, and coastal Guayaquil, the nation's largest city, to tiny clinics in Andean villages. We felt great about the free services we were providing to impoverished patients, some of whom walked for three days over mountain passes to bring their children for surgery. And then, as had happened two decades before in Culiacán, Mexico, we were kicked out of the country, for pretty much the same reasons: a small group of elite plastic surgeons felt our presence made them look bad.

This was a great blow to us and to one of our cherished partners and great boosters in Ecuador, Dr. Jorge

Palacios, a plastic and reconstructive surgeon who established his nation's first hospital burn unit. I met Jorge in 1977, when he spent three months at Stanford on a fellowship. That same year, I made my first trip to Ecuador. While we were there assessing patients for no-cost surgeries, I was asked to consult on a private case. The daughter of a wealthy businessman had been fed Drano by her psychotic babysitter. The little girl's whole mouth was burned on the inside. I was able to repair the damage with skin grafts. Her father, Faisal Misle, became an important supporter after that. He had invented a very lucrative knitting machine, and from then on, he donated half the proceeds from the device to needy patients.

I admired Jorge's energy, creativity, and compassion. Growing up, he told me, he'd wanted to be a fighter pilot. Then he read Albert Schweitzer's Nobel Peace Prize lecture and decided to become a healer, not a warrior. Jorge graduated with a degree in medicine and surgery from the University of Guayaquil and specialized in plastic surgery at the Ramos Mejía Hospital in Buenos Aires, Argentina. He'd originally planned on being a cardiovascular surgeon and hoped to be the first Ecuadorian to perform a heart transplant. But one day when he was an intern on call, he treated a deeply depressed patient who'd attempted suicide with an overdose of Valium. After a stomach-pumping, the man was unconscious, so Jorge asked his wife for basic information. "Then," he told me, "she took out her wallet and showed me a picture of a beautiful girl of about seventeen. 'She is the reason why my husband is like he is now.' I didn't want to ask questions in case the young woman was a mistress or something like that. The woman told me to come back to her husband's room at three in the afternoon, and she would explain." Intrigued by the mystery, Jorge showed up — and met the girl in the photo, now terribly disfigured by burns to her face and body, injuries sustained when someone threw a Molotov cocktail at their passing car during a protest.

"This man, her father, could not accept the suffering of his only daughter," Jorge said. "I thought about how I could help her, and that's when I thought of plastic surgery. I could see how plastic surgery could fix this thing that is destroyed, but still I said to myself, *I want to be a cardiovascular surgeon.* I didn't want to change my objective, so it was a fight in my mind." Jorge went on to train in both cardiovascular surgery and plastic surgery — but he had found his true calling.

In 1986, not long after Jorge established the first burn unit in Ecuador, at Luis Vernaza Hospital in Guayaquil, he was refused admission to the Ecuadorian Society of Plastic Surgeons for, as Jorge put it, "consorting with gringos." The president of the society and some of his colleagues believed the success of Interplast reflected poorly on the work they were doing. We were encroaching on their territory and showing them up. Not only did they want to bar Jorge from their society because he had arranged for Interplast to enter the country, they wanted us gone.

Luckily, Jorge happened to be married to a former Miss Ecuador, who happened to be friends with María Eugenia

Cordovez, the wife of the president of the republic. The first lady appealed to her husband, León Febres Cordero, to reinstate Interplast and suggested he do so by awarding me the nation's highest honor, the Medal of Merit. The president agreed, and his head of protocol called me to say that ceremony was set for two weeks hence. He also told me that the president would expect a gift in return. I asked what the last recipient of the Medal of Merit had given the president. It was a thoroughbred racehorse.

I did some research and discovered that the president was a pistol-shooting champion. Friends in Ecuador agreed that presenting him with some coveted firearm — much cheaper than a racehorse — was a great idea. I asked a Stanford colleague, a cardiac surgeon who's a gun fancier, what I should bring. "Oh," he said, "you've got to give him the Gun That Won the West — the Kentucky long rifle, Daniel Boone's weapon of choice. There are only five of them in existence, and I can lay my hands on one. I can get it to you in three or four weeks." It would only cost me $10,000. I gulped and said I appreciated his help, but I had to be in Ecuador in two weeks.

Next, I turned to a friend who's an avid hunter. He said, "Well, Don, this is the perfect opportunity to give him the Gun That Won the West."

"But I can't get that rifle in time, and it's ten thousand bucks!" I said.

"No, no — not a rifle," he said. "I mean the Colt 45. The Gun That Won the West! I'm a licensed dealer so I can get one for you at a good price, but it will take a few weeks." I thanked him and started to panic.

I mentioned my problem to the scrub nurse at my next surgery. "Oh, my husband can help you," she said. "He's president of Ducks Unlimited, and he's into firearms." She called him and reported back to me. "He can get you the Gun That Won the West!" she said.

"I've tried two of those," I told her.

"No, this is *really* the Gun That Won the West — the Winchester repeating rifle, and he can get you one right away for $200." She brought it in the next day. Then I called a friend who'd worked for a secret government organization — okay, the CIA — to find out how to get the gun out of the country. He told me that I had to alert Eastern Airlines in advance, then put the gun in a box with hard sides, affix a form from the airlines to the box, and carry a letter signed by a lawyer or a notary saying that I'd been invited by the president of Ecuador.

I showed up at the airport for a red-eye, wearing a pork-pie hat, dark glasses, and a leather bomber jacket. I gave my name at the counter, and the reservation agent looked me up in the computer. Her jaw dropped. "It says you're carrying a gun!" I assured her that I'd taken the proper steps, and everything went the way it was supposed to.

The president loved the Gun That Won the West. The best part? The man he'd asked to bestow the Medal of Merit at a public ceremony was the president of the Ecuadorian Society of Plastic Surgeons, the very fellow who'd engineered our ouster. Not long after that, Jorge Palacios was accepted into the society. And Interplast, now ReSurge International, serves Ecuador to this day.

ELEVEN

THE ROLLS-ROYCE VAGINA AND THE POSTMODERN PENIS

By the late '80s, even after I'd been doing gender confirmation surgeries for twenty years, the surgical details of gender metamorphosis remained as fascinating to me as the social and political factors. Maybe more so. From the first, I was especially intrigued by the challenge of making sure people with gender dysphoria who sought surgery ended up with healthy, aesthetically pleasing new genitals that brought them psychological comfort and erotic satisfaction. To that end, I spent a good deal of the last quarter of the twentieth century creating or perfecting novel surgical procedures.

The penile-inversion vaginas, like the one I gave my first transgender patient, Ella, are fine and functional.

The procedure, developed by gender surgery pioneer Dr. Georges Burou in Casablanca, takes four to five hours in the hands of an experienced surgeon. It involves forming space between the rectum and the bladder and inverting the penis — essentially turning it inside out like a sock — and using the skin of the penis and sometimes skin grafts from the scrotum to line the vaginal vault. The testicles are removed, and scrotal skin is used to make the labia majora. The nerves and skin of the glans penis — the sensitive tip — are used to make a clitoris. The urethra is shortened, and sensitive urethral mucosa is placed in between the labia minora, the inner folds of the vagina. The cost, safety, and efficacy for this surgery compare with other major rehabilitation projects such as organ transplant or joint replacement. And the patients' positive responses upped my psychic income. I was able to contribute a helpful addition to the preparation for the procedure: before the surgery, the patient must undergo permanent hair removal in the genital area. I began using a type of X-ray called beta, which penetrates the skin a mere millimeter and does little damage.

Back in 1972, four years after I had performed my very first gender confirmation surgery, I operated on a patient I'll call Regina, the most beautiful trans woman I've ever seen. Our gender identity committee approved her for surgery after a one-year trial period; she'd been doing well on the female hormones progesterone and estrogen, and she had the support of family and friends. First, she had an augmentation mammoplasty with silicone implants. Then came penile-inversion vaginoplasty, with bed rest for seven days afterward so the skin grafts would heal properly. During that week, a dilator in the vaginal vault was inflated and deflated periodically to make sure the vaginal space remained concave. This intermittent dilation continued for six months to a year after the surgery. Regina was very happy with the results of her surgery.

"Magnificent!" declared Georges Burou, who examined Regina when he came to Stanford for our second international gender dysphoria symposium.

In the late 1980s, I began performing a different kind of vaginoplasty — rectosigmoid vaginoplasty, which resulted in what was nicknamed the "Rolls-Royce vagina," meant to be an improvement over the safe, serviceable "Volkswagen vagina," as one wag dubbed the penile-inversion procedure. The operation involves removing the penis and using a three- to four-inch section of the sigmoid colon — the part of the colon (also called the bowel or large intestine) closest to the anus and rectum — to create the vaginal vault. The section is harvested as a pedicle flap, with its nerve and blood supply intact, through an abdominal incision. Then the rest of the colon is reconnected, and the pedicle is put in place using scrotal skin flaps that also serve to create labia. As in penile-inversion vaginoplasty, the tip of the penis is used to form a clitoris. The surgery lasts six to seven hours.

Rectosigmoid vaginoplasty increases vaginal depth and creates a self-lubricating vagina that doesn't require postoperative dilation. Patients feel orgasms created by the stimulation of nerves that previously belonged to the prostate gland. Disadvantages of the procedure include the additional risks that accompany abdominal surgery, greater expense, and the possibility that the colon graft might, in rare cases, produce too much lubrication — excessive mucous discharge. This latter problem usually resolves within three to six months.

A 2015 article in the *Journal of Sexual Medicine* reviewed the outcomes of both types of vaginoplasty, as reported in twenty-six studies covering 1,461 patients who'd had penile-inversion surgery and 102 patients who'd had recto-sigmoid vaginoplasty. The incidence of complications, the general outcome, and the level of patient satisfaction were deemed comparable.

And in 2016, in the journal *Plastic and Reconstructive Surgery*, I, along with one of my former Stanford residents, Thomas Satterwhite, MD; Judy Van Maasdam, the longtime director of the Gender Dysphoria Program; and others published a study of safety and efficacy of recto-sigmoid vaginoplasty that followed up on eighty-three of my patients over twenty-two years. We conducted direct inquiries to determine the patients' levels of satisfaction with appearance, sexual function, and ease of postoperative recovery. Overall, the patients were healthy and happy. Forty-eight patients had complications, but over 80 percent of those complications were minor ones. (Smokers had higher complication rates.) Excessive mucous discharge occurred in 28.6 percent of patients in the majority of those cases but resolved after the first year. Patient satisfaction with appearance and sexual function was high.

Thomas Satterwhite, who was an outstanding resident, is now part of a surgical practice in Marin County, California, specializing in gender confirmation surgery. He's been kind enough to publicly acknowledge Judy Van Maasdam and me as early mentors. He observed in a recent newspaper interview that after gender confirmation surgery, patients formerly suffering from gender dysphoria report almost instantly experiencing a profound sense of life improvement — physically, emotionally, and spiritually.

One of the patients who benefited from the Rolls-Royce vagina was Molly, a New York venture capitalist. I remember that she had a follow-up exam scheduled as the last appointment of what had turned out to be a tough day. I'd seen several cosmetic surgery patients in a row who'd had excellent outcomes but were pestering me for further procedures to fulfill their futile pursuit for perfection. Getting them to listen to reason had been a lengthy and exhausting process and more contentious than I'd hoped.

When I finally got to Molly, we greeted each other warmly. I sighed and said, "I'm so glad to finally see a normal patient today, Molly." She lit up. "Thank you, Doctor. That's the first time anybody has ever called me normal!"

Some of my patients were trans men who wanted a penis after the requisite time spent on androgens — male-typical hormones — and a mastectomy if they desired it.

In early phalloplasties, the shape wasn't great; the shafts were too cigar-like (and early on I was accused by a female colleague of making them too big. A guy thing?).

But as I refined the surgery, the results got better and better. What I call the postmodern phalloplasty requires tremendous commitment on the part of the patient, who must devote six weeks to the process and undergo two procedures. Surgery takes place after at least a year of treatment with androgens.

First, the surgeon makes two vertical incisions four and a half inches apart in the lower abdomen. Then the surgeon lifts up a flap of skin and soft tissue, still attached at the ends, and rolls the fat and skin into a tube between the navel and bikini line. This is the new penis. The tube, which will form an internal tunnel for the urethra, is covered with a bandage and left to grow on the abdomen for six weeks, until it develops its own blood supply. The patient, meanwhile, is free to go about his life, with what looks like a sausage strapped tightly to his abdomen.

Step two is detaching the top of the tube forming the head of the penis and permitting the new organ to drop down. Erotic sensation is maintained by a sensory nerve that's transferred from the forearm to the tube of the neopenis and reconnected to the brain when it's microsurgically attached to the original erotic nerve in the abdomen, which formerly served the clitoris and now sensitizes the tip of the new penis. The placement of a removable silicone urinary assist device allows urination in the standing position. For erections, the multidisciplinary team adds either a permanent implant in the form of a bendable rod or a pump device inflated externally, or a removable rod inserted in the penis just before intercourse. To create a scrotum, surgeons insert skin expanders — little deflated balloons that we inflate bit by bit to stretch the skin — in the labia. The labia are sewn together, and after several weeks of expansion, we insert testicular implants — silicone balls.

I invented another less elaborate and less expensive procedure for transgender men, called a metoidioplasty (from *meta*, for change, and *oidio*, ancient Greek slang for male genitalia). This reconstructive surgery involves creating a small penis — about the size of a middle finger — from the testosterone-enlarged clitoris.

I was delighted to discover that genital surgery afforded the reconstructive surgeon additional opportunity to improve lives. Procedures that we initially developed for gender confirmation surgery have proved applicable to a variety of problems such as vaginal atresia, a condition in which the vagina is abnormally closed or absent; some types of dyspareunia (painful intercourse); and congenital adrenal hyperplasia, overdevelopment of genitalia caused when the adrenal gland of a developing female fetus produces extra androgens.

Of course, the new field of gender confirmation surgery attracted a few charlatans. In 1977, I testified as an expert witness at a hearing against the world's worst gender confirmation surgeon, John Ronald Brown, also known as Table-Top Brown because he often operated outside of hospitals or clinics. The California Board of Medical Quality Assurance took away Brown's license to practice medicine because of "gross negligence, incompetence, and practicing unprofessional medicine in a manner which involved moral turpitude." Among his many crimes: failing to hospitalize a patient with life-threatening complications; allowing an employee who wasn't a physician to perform surgery; skipping psychological screening, collecting of medical histories, and pre-op exams; and purposely damaging the vagina of a patient who angered him. His lack of surgical skills was appalling, as was his disregard for patient safety — Bay Area plastic surgeons often had to repair his shoddy work. After his license was revoked, he continued to practice without one in Tijuana, Mexico. In 1998, he was convicted of second-degree murder when one of his patients died in the U.S. after surgery south of the border — not a trans person, as it happened, but a fellow with a fetish called amputee identity disorder, the compulsion to have a healthy limb removed. Brown died in 2010 while serving a life sentence in California's Salinas Valley State Prison.

There were subtler ways to hurt patients seeking gender confirmation surgery. While Norman Fisk and I and our colleagues were successfully treating gender dysphoria, a vocal physician at the very institution that had pioneered the work was insisting that surgical intervention for gender dysphoria was not just ineffective but morally dangerous, despite evidence to the contrary. Johns Hopkins made big news when it became the first university to perform gender confirmation surgery in 1966. In 1979, it made news again when the Johns Hopkins Gender Identity Clinic was shut down by Paul

McHugh, then the university's psychiatrist-in-chief, on the grounds that the surgery was "promoting a mental disorder" and that it failed to improve the lives of patients. He based that conclusion on a single widely discredited 1977 follow-up study of fifty trans people who underwent surgery at Johns Hopkins. The study concluded that gender confirmation surgery confers no "social rehabilitation" for trans people. Johns Hopkins resumed gender confirmation surgery in April 2017. I'm pained when I think about the unnecessary heartache caused by this nearly four-decade ban.

TWELVE

THE CAST OF CHARACTERS
(AND CHARACTERS IN CASTS)

I'd need several volumes to chronicle the extraordinary humans I've met during my years of practice on this planet. I've already introduced some of them, but I want to share my experiences with a few more outstanding characters: Clair the Tattooed Millionairess, Dutch the Motorhead, Tacho the Spy, Pancho the Kiwi King, and a noted physician/writer who felt himself to be the victim of intellectual property theft.

One day in the mid-1960s — before I'd dreamed of Interplast or even knew about gender dysphoria — after working thirty-six hours straight, I was grabbing a snack in the cafeteria when I heard my name over the hospital loudspeaker. I was to report to the emergency room, stat. "You're late, Doctor!" the nurse said. "Do the H&P [history and physical] on the incarcerated hernia in room three." When an experienced nurse pronounces "Doctor" with the first syllable going up and the second syllable going down without saying your last name, you know that the nurse is really saying "shithead." I quickly reviewed the chart for *Clair Elgin, age 60, room 3, acute abdomen* . . . and hopped into room 3, where I saw a large woman in pain. I introduced myself, and she told me that after breakfast the previous day, she'd experienced some cramps that got worse; she'd vomited and hadn't had a bowel movement since then. The pain was in her lower right side. She lifted her hospital gown, and I felt for tenderness that would indicate possible inflammatory appendicitis, or rebound tenderness, which would indicate a rupture of the appendix and peritonitis. I didn't feel either. But in her groin, I felt a lump about an inch in diameter. Her abdomen was distended, and I percussed her distended abdomen and detected a lot of gas in there. I also observed that every square inch of the skin that I had just seen was tattooed in a rather intricate and lovely floral and filigree pattern.

I did a rectal exam and tested the stool for blood. There wasn't any. "It looks like you're going to need surgery to find out exactly what's going on here," I told Clair. "You may have a hernia — a loop of bowel stuck down there." She thought a minute, then asked, "Doctor, where do you make the incision?" I showed her. She said, "If you possibly can, be sure to get that tattoo realigned exactly when you do the suturing."

The excellent Dr. Ed Hurley, a young cardiac surgeon in training who'd be assisting in the exploratory surgery, had entered the room and heard Clair's request. "Dr. Laub wants to be a plastic surgeon," he said, "so that'll be his job." He left the room.

I started an IV while attempting small talk with Clair, which went nowhere. Then she said, "Doctor, there's something you should know. Please keep it quiet. People in general are not aware that I originally had a penis." I replied, still attempting lightness, "Well, I don't see it here. What did you do with it?"

"I didn't want it," she said, "so I removed it myself because I couldn't get any surgeon to do it." Looking back a few years later, I realized that Clair Elgin was actually my first trans patient, though of a very unusual sort.

Clair told me her story. She was born in Saudi Arabia, the son of a Muslim woman and a Scottish trader who ran a ship between Arabia and England, and she was educated aboard a ship by world-class tutors. She was genetically XY and was born with hypospadias, a birth defect that causes urine to come out just above the scrotum. Because this deformity made Clair's genitalia appear to be a clitoris and labia, her parents assumed she was a girl and raised her as one. No genetic testing was available to them at the time. When Clair reached puberty, she developed an ample penis, which was understandably upsetting for her. For many years, she told me, she'd unsuccessfully sought medical help. She moved to Los Angeles. Unable to live as the woman she felt she was, she removed her penis and testicles with a sharp knife and presented herself at the University of California emergency room. Notable urologist Dr. Willard Goodwin, who was sympathetic to her plight, took her as his patient and fixed her up to the degree that was possible at the time.

Now, at Stanford Hospital, Clair was put under the care of Dr. Harry A. Oberhelman, a professor of surgery specializing in the gastrointestinal tract. I was to scrub in on the surgery as second assistant, and I was quite excited at the chance to learn about an incarcerated inguinal hernia — a piece of intestine protruding through a weak spot in the abdominal wall, blocking the blood supply that intestinal tissue needs to stay alive.

As we worked, Dr. Hurley explained the pathophysiology of the incarcerated hernia: the testicles in a male's embryonic life originally enjoy a home around the kidneys. Shortly before birth, under the influence of hormonal signals, they descend through the groin area into the area of the external genitalia. In effect, these masses of germinal tissue called testicles end up in the labia, which become enlarged and assume the role of the scrotum. Occasionally, the bowel follows the testicle down, and if the passageway hasn't spontaneously closed before birth, an incipient hernia is produced. Clair Elgin was in danger of dying because the intestine's blood supply can be easily blocked off by the swollen tissues.

Dr. Hurley deftly made the incision and dissected expertly down to the loop of bowel that formed the lump. With manual pressure, gentle yet firm, he coaxed the incarcerated segment of large intestine back into its rightful home in the abdominal cavity. Clair's hernia was reduced just in time because the bowel segment had begun to turn cyanotic blue, the sign that it was dying from lack of arterial blood flow. When the intestine was liberated from the lump, it pinked up as circulation was restored. Clair was out of danger.

As Dr. Hurley was closing the bowel incision, I told him what Clair had revealed about her sex. He simply said, "Oh." As promised, I sutured the skin extra carefully to preserve the integrity of Clair's tattoo art as much as possible.

She healed well and was a most pleasant patient. Her face and feet weren't tattooed, but most everything else was. On the back of each elbow was an eye. When she straightened her arms, the eye closed. I asked her about her body art, and she told me she'd once traveled with a circus as a tattooed lady and sword swallower. She was interesting and nice, so I made a place for her in my mental list of friends. I was glad that her recovery went so well.

When Clair left the hospital, my duty as an intern was to make a discharge summary, putting all the facts of the case on one typed page. In her chart, I noted that in the urinalysis I'd ordered, there was microscopic evidence of the presence of red blood cells. I called and asked her to come in and repeat the test. Again, it was positive for red blood cells. Then we ordered an intravenous pyelogram (IVP), an X-ray taken with dye infused into the kidney by way of a vein in the arm. Clair was compliant, although naturally wondering why we were concerned. I was as helpful as I could be without mentioning the

C-word. The IVP turned up a hypernephroma, a type of kidney cancer. I explained the condition to Clair and told her that she needed to have the left kidney surgically removed. Dr. Oberhelman performed a brilliant operation. Again, Clair made a fine recovery.

As I made daily rounds, I noticed a frequent visitor to Clair's room: a man with a stiff leg, indicating a knee fusion, and a pirate's chest worth of flashy jewelry, including a huge gold cross on a chain, diamond rings, and an unusually large ring featuring the words *ménage à trois* etched in amber. His typical outfit was an orange jumpsuit (non-prison style). After a few days, I asked Clair who he was.

Gene Gaynor, she told me, was her "private nurse." He'd been an army nurse, running a military hospital OR in Fiji and in Korea during the war. He'd fractured his leg when he was accompanying wounded combatants from Korea to Japan, and their plane crashed into a mountain. Because he was sitting next to a door that blew open, hurling him into a mound of snow, he was the only person who didn't perish. After his rescue, he was brought stateside to the VA hospital in Los Angeles, where he was scheduled for above-the-knee amputation of his left leg. He refused the surgery. He was still in the hospital, attempting to heal his knee and not doing well when Clair met him. She was a Pink Lady at the VA, entertaining patients by coming around and playing tunes on her harmonica. Clair felt sorry for Gene and hired him as her factotum and, when necessary, nurse. The relationship was strictly professional.

Clair was an intriguing bundle of habits, interests, and skills. Having been raised Muslim, she abstained from drinking alcohol. She owned a motorcycle, a Gullwing Mercedes, and an expensive telescopic rifle. Her profession was photography, which she had been taught on her father's ship by a tutor. In the early days of Silicon Valley, she was involved in developing ways to use microphotography as part of the manufacturing of computer chips, which earned her a large number of shares in a laser and computer company that later became wildly successful. Clair loved Japanese architecture, and with her money, she built a Japanese home — a five-sided pagoda with a vista in Los Altos Hills, not far from Stanford. The design included koi ponds that allowed the fish to swim from outside her home to inside. The five alcoves of the pagoda each had a wind-driven pipe organ that Clair enjoyed playing. Gene lived in a separate house on the side of the hill.

I essentially became Clair's general practitioner, treating sore throats, colds, constipation, and other minor things. I always kept Dr. Oberhelman informed about Clair's health. I had begun seeing patients in Mexico, in the program that became Interplast, and I showed Clair before and after pictures of patients with cleft lips and palates and burn scars. She was very touched by what she saw.

I treated Clair when she came to the hospital after an infection left severe tendon scarring in her right index finger. She was hospitalized under the care of Robert Chase, who treated her with skillful surgery. Still, Clair ended up with a stiff finger, which meant she couldn't play the organ. After that, she depended on another of Gene's talents. He had been trained as a concert pianist, and in the army, he'd been called upon to provide background music for top-brass cocktail parties.

As time passed Clair began to complain to me about a dry cough and intermittent pneumonia. She had a history of heavy smoking, so we needed to check for lung cancer. Indeed, that was the problem. And it was solved; the tumor was successfully irradiated and eradicated.

Not long after that, Clair again desired surgery, this time to improve her appearance. The many lines in her face made her look more male than female. We did a face-lift, which went very well. After the face-lift, in a follow-up visit, when the time seemed right psychologically, I showed Clair more photos of patients in Mexico and said, "Clair, I'm not very good at asking people for money, but I was hoping that you might donate $3,000 to our Mexico project, because you seem quite interested in those kids."

She looked at me, surprised and amused, and said, "Well, you're the most goddamned ungrateful person I've ever known! I just changed my will to leave you three million dollars. And now you're asking me for three thousand more?"

I was stunned. "Clair!" I said. "I'm so sorry! I don't know anything about any three million dollars. Who did you give it to?"

"I arranged it with the dean. It's for Dr. Oberhelman's cancer research and for your Mexico project."

I thanked her profusely and went rampaging down

the hall. I ran into Dr. Oberhelman, told him what Clair had said, and declared that the dean was planning to steal our money. "I'm pretty angry about it," I said, "and I'm going there right now to ask him for it!"

"Watch it!" Dr. Oberhelman warned. "You don't have tenure yet — he may fire you on the spot!"

"Yes, he can do that," I said. "But what he's doing is unethical and immoral. I'll be back."

The dean's secretary looked a bit alarmed when I entered his office. "I'm Dr. Laub," I said, "and I'd like to see the dean right away."

"May I tell him what it's about?"

"Money."

"One moment."

She went into the dean's office, then came back, saying, "The dean's behind closed doors and can't see you now."

"This is urgent. When can he see me?"

"I don't know."

"Okay," I said. "Let me see the person in charge of development."

She checked his office and returned. "The dean is busy."

I calmed myself. "Please do me a favor, if you would be so kind," I said. "Check the file on Clair Elgin. See if it says something interesting or peculiar that may have something to do with me, Dr. Donald Laub."

She did as I asked, holding the file protectively close to her chin. As she scanned the pages slowly and carefully, her eyes widened, and her expression changed. I had finally gotten her attention.

"Oh. Oh, yes." She then went into the dean's office and came right back. "The dean will see you now."

I explained to the dean that Ms. Elgin had donated $3 million to Dr. Oberhelman and me, but we hadn't been informed. He looked uncomfortable. "Oh, yes," he said. "I must admit we diverted Ms. Elgin's bequest to general funds. That's the way willed gifts to the university work."

I said, "That's *my* money!"

The dean said he thought he could get me $10,000 right away. In a few days, another administrator, the associate dean for special gifts, called me to say, "I've got $10,000 for you and Dr. Oberhelman. You should feel very happy about that."

I told all this to Dr. Oberhelman the next day in the locker room as we dressed for surgery. Despite what the dean told us we *should* feel, neither of us was happy about what had transpired. Eventually, we accepted it, though we were still indignant at the injustice. One day I said, "Harry, we've saved Clair Elgin's life a couple of times, and I've given her a face-lift. We've taken good care of her. And the dean took her $3 million and gave us $10,000. I think we should go to her home and ask her to change her bequest."

"We may get into trouble," he said.

"Then let's get into trouble," I said.

So, we made an appointment with Clair. Gene Gaynor welcomed us and asked us to take our shoes off, Japanese-style. We complied and admired the koi ponds. Clair came out, invited us to sit down, and offered us coffee.

Gene played a few tunes on one of Clair's five organs. The music was loud, genuine, and wonderful.

Clair asked why we had come over. We explained what had happened with the dean and her gift and said that we thought we deserved the money she wanted to leave us. We were there to ask her to change her will.

"I can handle this with a simple phone call," she said. She picked up a red telephone on the desk that had a direct connection to Jack, her lawyer. She asked him to change her will so that Dr. Oberhelman and I were the beneficiaries. "When it's ready," she told Jack, "I'll drive my motorcycle down and sign it."

We were overjoyed, and Clair was pleased. Harry and I barreled back to Stanford and burst into Dr. Chase's office as I yelled, "Boss, we just made three million bucks!" Sitting on Chase's couch was the dean. "Where have you boys been this morning?" he asked. "Up at Clair Elgin's, by any chance?"

Our hearts sank. We figured we were fired. But we owned up to the visit. "Yes," I said, "we've just come from there."

"Well, you shouldn't have done that," the dean said. "But you do deserve the money. It was the best thing to do." We were feeling great again.

A few months later, Gene asked to have a private conference with me. Clair was feeling down, he reported, and doing nothing but using her newfangled video recorder to tape her favorite shows — especially *Columbo* — and then watching them during the day. She was drinking coffee and smoking all night, and she had intermittent pulmonary problems. Gene didn't know how to make Clair feel better. I thought about the situation for two days and came up with the idea of making Clair the official Interplast photographer. She loved the idea and brightened up considerably.

Clair made numerous trips to Central and South America with Interplast teams, taking pictures to chronicle surgeries for cleft lip, cleft palate, and burn scar deformities. She was greatly appreciated for the excellence of her photography and her compassion toward patients. In Latin America, patients called her "Señor Clair," and didn't seem to care a whit about her gender.

During the era of the Interplast Airforce, Clair also served as a human altimeter; our DC-3 wasn't pressurized, so every time we flew above 3,000 feet, she'd fall asleep and start turning blue.

Gene came on several Interplast trips, too, and though he wasn't the most socially adept person, he proved a great asset. One night in San Pedro Sula, Honduras, for example, the operating room was flooded with sewage. Gene got up at 4 a.m., put on his big boots, got a mop, and cleaned up the whole mess. He was totally committed.

Time passed, and Gene came to see me again. He said Clair's fortunes had sunk in the recession of the 1970s. She was bankrupt, and all the money in reserve for Interplast and cancer was no more. Clair had become despondent again, and Gene asked if I could think up another worthwhile thing for her to do, since the Interplast photography had worked out so well. "Gene," I said, "how can I ever think of something else?" But Gene pushed. "Come on, boy, you're the colonel. You've got to think." So about four days later, I came up with the idea that Clair should invent 3-D television. And she did, protecting her invention with overlapping patents and forming a company. She sold the hilltop pagoda complex, and she and Gene moved into a modest home in Redwood City, where they lived happily until one Saturday morning when she called me.

"Doctor, I have severe pain in the rib when I cough. It came on suddenly." On the phone, I was able to determine that the pain, located in a single part of one rib, was probably caused by a pathologic fracture — one that occurs without trauma. Often it signals a metastasis from cancer of the lung to the bone. I drove to her house and put my finger where the pain was. It felt tender and mushy. I knew what was probably going on.

A physician on duty at Stanford Hospital agreed to admit Clair immediately to the oncology medical service. There weren't many senior doctors around on the weekend, but an intern would provide competent care.

When I brought Clair to the hospital, however, I found that the experienced intern was off for the weekend as well, and the person in charge was a very newly minted MD. This was, in fact, her first serious case. I debriefed her in detail and said that it was likely to be cancer. She asked what I would advise. I told her she should certainly tell the patient whatever was found, but she could also say that more radiation therapy might be possible, that new drugs are always around the corner, that you can never tell if there will be a cure from some novel and peculiar regimen. Be rather upbeat about it all, I said.

The intern said no. She had decided early in her career that she would always be honest with the patient. If there was a cancer, she would tell the patient the truth about that cancer. I suggested that it was possible to be honest and still preserve hope. She disagreed. So be it, I thought, and I went home.

Over the weekend, chest and rib X-rays showed that Clair's lung cancer had metastasized to the rib. The young doctor marched into Clair's room with the X-ray in hand and showed her the cancer.

"Oh?" Clair said. "What kind of cancer?"

"Well, it's metastatic cancer, probably from that cancer of the lung you had before."

Clair was ready with the next question. "Doctor, how long do you think I have to live?"

"I'd say about six weeks. You really ought to get your things in order."

"I see. Thanks very much for telling me so precisely. Doctor, would you mind giving me a glass of water?" The intern did so. "And would you mind handing me my purse?" Clair opened it and took out a little package. It contained cyanide capsules. She swallowed one, had a seizure, and keeled over. The young doctor desperately resuscitated Clair, who breathed for twenty-four hours more. But she was essentially gone the minute she swallowed the cyanide.

The young doctor called to inform me, and I was absolutely furious with her. I yelled, "I told you not to do that. Look what you've done!" She stammered some answer I can't remember.

I was terrifically upset that a medical student on her first case had done something that I wouldn't do. After the passage of several decades, however, I began to think that perhaps she was right. I remembered Clair asking, "Please tell me when I don't have long to live. I'd like to know so I can do something about it." I never really took that to heart, never heard what she was saying, or chose not to understand what "doing something about it" meant. But of course, she was saying that she planned to go out with a minimum of suffering. That was her free election. But I didn't catch it at the time.

By the end of Clair's life, there was no money left for Interplast. But she'd given something more precious. Clair was a friend, a patient, a coworker, an essential member of the team. She was dedicated, strange, valuable, loyal. She was a reminder to me that outliers often have great inner gifts and make wonderful friends.

Another patient who stands out in my memory is an avid motorcycle racer named Dutch, who reached for his shotgun during what he believed to be a break-in at the rural Northern California home he shared with his wife and children. He accidentally shot himself, splattering the skin and muscle of his left hand, fracturing the bones, and contaminating the wound with gunpowder and lead. Amazingly, the nerves and tendons were uninjured.

It was 1967, and I was in my fourth year of surgery training at Stanford, on a rotation at San Mateo County Hospital. When I met Dutch and his shattered paw in the emergency room, he told me he had one goal: being able to once again shift the clutch on his Harley with his left hand.

Fortunately, I'd had training in hand surgery from William Frackleton in medical school and Robert Chase as a resident, and I'd assisted Harry Buncke at Stanford. Furthermore, the attending physician on call at the hospital was the excellent Dr. Richard Gonzales, who was in practice with Buncke. Gonzales advised me to use a Baylor hand immobilizer, and we devised one for Dutch. This was an old technique, but it was new to me: each digit of the wounded hand was to be held outstretched and immobilized so the multiple fractures could heal. Rubber bands attached to the fingers with tape would pull the digits out toward a big hoop formed from thick, malleable copper wire and held in place with a plaster of Paris forearm cast. The device looked something like a jai-alai cesta — the basket-like device that jai-alai players use to catch and hurl the ball. Or maybe like an old-fashioned snowshoe.

Every week Dr. Gonzales and I reviewed new X-rays to check Dutch's progress and adjust the advice accordingly by moving the elastic bands. I was amazed by and pleased with the immobilizer; it was, if you'll pardon the pun, very handy.

When the threat of infection had cleared and the fractured fingers were healing, we detached Dutch from the immobilizer and began to transfer a flap of skin and nice fat from his abdomen. Dutch's hand was attached to his abdomen for three and a half weeks. We weaned the flap away from its nourishing blood supply on the abdomen by sequentially decreasing circulation using tourniquets, and then by operations to gradually close out the abdominal blood supply and force the tissue to gain new blood supply on both sides of the base of his hand. We placed bone grafts for stability of the hand and wrist bones; they healed on schedule and became solid.

It was a joyous day when Dutch showed up at the clinic in San Mateo for a post-rehabilitation follow-up riding his Harley. He invited me to sit on the rear seat and drove me around the block, shifting gears repeatedly with his left hand. It was heaven on wheels.

On our first morning in Culiacán, Sinaloa, Mexico, in the 1960s, Tacho, an unshaven man in raggedy clothes, came to the Interplast clinic complaining of mild facial palsy and asking for free treatment because he had no money. After we examined him and took his history, he remained in the clinic all day, observing.

Tacho later revealed that he was spying on us on behalf of the Colegio Médico, the local medical society, to see if we really were good people or just gringos with a clever angle on self-aggrandizement. He had no facial palsy, and he wasn't particularly poor; he lived in a comfortable house. He sold used car parts and other materials that he'd obtained when he worked doing demolition in Tijuana. A few years earlier, he'd contracted a testicular infection and almost died. He promised God that if he recovered, he'd give half of all his future earnings to the poor. He also let it be known around town that he would give a free meal to anyone who needed it and find them work.

Tacho became our fixer, supporter, and patient finder. Twice, he intervened as a lifesaver. The first time, we'd been invited to a Sunday afternoon *bautismo*, the baptismal party for a newborn, at his home. We ate great food, laughed a lot, and danced in a large tent. I cut in on multiple dancing couples, unaware that in the culture of Sinaloa, doing so is an insult to masculinity punishable by shooting. I cut in on a ninety-two-year-old man and began to dance with his partner. He pulled out a gold-plated revolver and began to shoot rounds through the roof of the tent. One of Tacho's servants wrestled him to the ground, and Tacho himself took the gun out of the man's hands. Cultural awareness achieved.

During another party at Tacho's farm compound, we discovered a Resusci Anne, the dummy upon which medical students practice CPR. She was lying on a cot at the edge of the property. We asked Tacho, "Do you teach CPR?"

"No," he said. "She is the bodyguard." We thought he was joking and left. But after midnight, David Dibbell and I had to trespass back onto Tacho's property in the dark because we had forgotten our fishing rods there. We passed the "bodyguard" on the cot, and I jokingly delivered a chest thump with my fist. The next thing I knew, Resusci Anne had put a pistol in my mouth. After hours, it turned out, the mannequin, meant to scare off intruders, was replaced by a real human bodyguard. All was explained, and all was forgiven.

When I visited Tacho's home with Judy, he took pleasure

in showing us various artworks and artifacts, including some souvenirs of the Mexican Revolution. We didn't know that all the pieces we admired and praised were being collected by a servant walking behind us, to be presented to us later as gifts. Judy politely refused most of them. But several months later, when Tacho came north and stayed with us in Palo Alto, he got up at 2 a.m. one night and hung all of those gifts on our wall with fishing line!

Francisco "Pancho" Martinez came into my life through a chain of friendship that illustrates one of my basic life principles: always talk to strangers. In the mid-1970s, we moved to a house on six acres in Los Altos Hills. I chatted regularly with the garbage man who visited our property weekly, Magdaleno, who had come to California from Jalisco, Mexico. He became my friend and then my patient. I performed surgery at no cost to him, a full-thickness skin graft to the palmar surface of his fingers — the flat side — which had peeled due to dermatitis.

One day Magdaleno appeared at my office with a friend of his from Jalisco, who, he said, needed my help. Pancho Martinez had a severe bilateral cleft lip and palate with significant nasal deformity. A shy fellow because of his condition, Pancho had been picking lemons in Ventura County, California, for eight years. I didn't need to ask Pancho why he'd come to see me, although I probably should have; asking the patient their explicit and unspoken agenda is something we physicians must never forget to do. Pancho bravely produced his will and his bank account, signifying that he was prepared to die on the operating table without burdening others with the cost of his burial. I scrutinized the documents respectfully and then offered him free surgery.

The operation went well; Pancho was very happy with his new face. Immediately after the surgery, he recuperated at the home of Magdaleno, who delivered him punctually to the clinic for follow-up visits. One afternoon, I brought Pancho over to our property to stroll around. He was very interested in our kiwi vines.

When Judy and the kids and I first moved to a house with a large plot of land in Los Altos Hills, we removed more than 300 acacia trees planted by the previous owner. (A friend well-versed in explosives dynamited the stumps, first covering them with coarse sand, then covering each stump in turn with a large, heavy blast blanket and blowing it up. It was a fascinating and seemingly endless operation.) Then I moonlighted as a Christmas tree farmer, planting our six acres with conifers, which we cared for as a family, assisted by various workers. I'd hoped to make some extra money for Interplast, but though the enterprise was fun, it wasn't terribly lucrative. Then one day I came across a magazine called *California Grape Grower*, for people in the table grape and wine industry, and saw an article about the hot new glamour crop: kiwifruit, formerly known by the unglamorous name Chinese gooseberry. You could plant kiwi and make money, the story said. I went home and said to Judy, "Honey, I have a great idea." Out went the Christmas trees and in went the kiwifruit vines. I hoped they would fatten Interplast's coffers.

The vines grew on trellises eight feet high, built from 24-by-12-inch posts sunk three and a half feet into concrete. Wires held the plants to the trellises, and the fruit hung down five and a half feet off the ground, just the right height for picking. Kiwifruit are dioecious — there are male and female plants. Only the female vines produce fruit — 500 fruits per vine, which we could sell for a buck apiece — and for a good yield, you need to plant eight female vines for every male. We planted 318 vines. Unfortunately, the grower who sold us the vines mixed up the males and females, and we couldn't tell them apart until they flowered — females have bright white blossoms and males have white blossoms with a brilliant yellow stigma — a stalk with a sticky little bulb — in the center. After that, we had to do some transplanting to get the vines correctly distributed — transgender surgery, you might say.

We acquired several beehives so the vines would be pollinated — another absorbing hobby. Our soil had too much clay, so we modified it with loads of composted horse manure that we picked up at Campbell's mushroom processing plant on the other side of the Santa Cruz Mountains, near the coastal town of Pescadero. The vines needed plenty of weeding with a rototiller.

Pancho looked with great interest at the blossoming vines, the weeds, the irrigation pipes we were laying. "Can you use a shovel and hoe?" I asked him in my fractured Spanish. He said, "*Con mucho gusto.*" I immediately hired Pancho as my special assistant, and he moved into a trailer on our property. Along with me, Judy, and our son

Ray, he became part of the team that drove our old green pickup to Pescadero and back, loaded high with compost and pulling a wooden trailer filled with even more. I figured out that over the life of our kiwifruit enterprise, the four of us made fifty-two trips. Sometimes I left at dawn since I needed to be back at Stanford at 7 a.m. for the first case of the day.

Pancho could dig drainage ditches and post holes with absolute precision. An exceptional worker, he also handled irrigation, weeding, pruning, picking, sorting the fruit by size, and boxing. The kids helped, deepening their already fine work ethic. I turned out to be allergic to kiwi fuzz, so I was spared picking and packing duties; Judy's brothers — the ones who'd given me their stamp of approval when we were teenagers — pitched in. We called our business the Kiwi Patch; the logo was a California quail chasing a kiwi bird. This was one of the many schemes of mine that survived on wife support: Judy was in charge of selling, delivering, and billing. We sold the kiwis successfully to restaurants, fruit markets, and wholesalers.

Now that his cleft lip and palate were repaired, Pancho set out to find a wife. He corresponded with a woman in his hometown who agreed to marry him. Rita had one leg shorter than the other, Pancho said, but she was "very beautiful." He fitted out the green truck with a camper top, put a mattress in there, and fixed it all up nicely for his triumphant trip home to pick up his new bride.

When Pancho got to Jalisco, however, Rita changed her mind. On the drive home, he stopped in Tijuana and assuaged his sorrows with ecstasy, after which he lost a week of his life and all of his hair (I assume his baldness was a result of the toxicity of the drugs he was taking). He showed up at our house much the worse for wear. He started drinking too much beer and one night ran the green truck off the road. Then he disappeared. When we finally located him, we learned that he'd spent time in jail.

Back with us, he brightened up with some hard work. Eventually, Pancho met and married Lidia, a good woman who'd been a strawberry picker. She moved into the trailer on our property and became pregnant. She had terrible morning sickness, and her dehydration from vomiting was so severe that I set her up with an IV infusion in the trailer. Pancho changed the IV bottles and cared for her. All worked well. Gradually the nausea dissipated, and she gave birth to Johnny Juan, a chubby, charming kid.

When Judy and the kids and I moved to another property nearby, I gave Pancho my used Cadillac. He and Lidia loaded it to the ceiling and set off to San Angelo, Texas. Pancho used his savings to buy four apartment buildings. Judy gave Johnny Juan a $500 U.S. savings bond for his second birthday, to which we further contributed every year. Using that money as his tuition, Johnny Juan earned a master's degree in kinesiology where they parlayed his wages into ownership of four more apartment buildings

Pancho and I enriched each other's lives and those of our families. We all found value in manual labor. We nurtured Johnny Juan, a superb world citizen. That's the payoff when you talk to strangers.

The kiwifruit farm ultimately succumbed to gophers; they found the vines' roots delicious and gobbled them up, no matter what anti-rodent strategies we tried. When we moved to our new place, we planted 15,000 palm trees.

One final anecdote that amuses me: the late Richard Selzer, a surgeon who left medicine for literature, joined an Interplast mission to Arequipa, Peru, in 1984. He was good fun, but his ego took up a lot of space. I told him the story of Salvador — how the Mexicali team had repaired his cleft lip after he died on the operating table so we could fulfill his mother's dream of his meeting God with a perfect smile. The next year a fictionalized account of the event, the short story "Imelda," appeared in Selzer's book *Letters to a Young Doctor*. The story became immensely popular, and Selzer later said, "That happened, sort of." I didn't mind his using the material for fiction. But then a funny thing happened a few years later. I happened to treat a child who'd been in an accident. The patient's father wrote for the TV medical drama *Chicago Hope*. We often chatted during the course of his kid's treatment. I told him about Salvador and the perfect smile — and a version of the story made its way onto *Chicago Hope*. In the episode, one of the surgeon characters, seeking a consult on a new procedure, even said he was going to "call Don Laub at Stanford." After the show aired, I got an indignant call from Selzer. "Can you believe it?" he said. "They stole my story! I should sue!"

THIRTEEN

THE OLD ORDER CHANGETH

At the end of the 1990s, Interplast underwent some institutional upheavals that were probably inevitable but tough on me — big shifts in the makeup of the board, the goals of the organization, and my role in it.

Updating the board of directors made sense. For nearly three decades, the Interplast board had been made up almost entirely of medical professionals; surgeons ran the show. I understood that, for fundraising purposes, it was time to open the board to more businessfolk, and we welcomed some Silicon Valley heavyweights — executives from companies such as Google, Oracle, and Cisco Systems.

At the turn of the millennium, competition for donor dollars was intense. In 1968, Interplast was the only organization providing free reconstructive surgery in the developing world. By 1999, 104 organizations were delivering similar services. In 1968, my dream had been that someday 25 percent of all American plastic and reconstructive surgeons would have participated in international humanitarian surgical trips. By 2000, that number was 70 percent. The more the merrier, I thought. The newly constituted board, however, worried that not only was the donor pool diminishing, so was the volunteer pool. Still, Interplast had more than 2,500 volunteer doctors and nurses from all over the U.S. We were visiting thirty countries and performing more than 3,000 surgeries each year.

I understood that Interplast's success meant we had to professionalize the administration, and to that end, the board filled the newly created positions of CEO and medical director — with a plastic surgeon who wasn't me. The new CEO put in place strict rules for every aspect of carrying out Interplast's medical missions. I told her that the high quality of the people I chose to lead missions was better than a rule. You have to make tough split-second decisions operating in a foreign country, and the trip leader should have total control over that decision-making. You don't need a rule book if the team is top-notch, I said. Interplast isn't about rules — it's about spirit.

The new board agreed with the CEO. Its members also called for more attention to the bottom line and clearer metrics so we could show donors exactly what they were getting for their money. The way I heard it was, Don, you're running this thing like a nutty doctor; we need to run it like a business. The board declared that

I was making too many decisions myself, that I refused to stick to an agenda, that I thrived on chaos. I would have added a couple of modifiers: productive, creative chaos.

The board proposed two changes I found particularly disheartening and wrongheaded: no longer bringing residents and interns on trips and recalibrating Interplast's mission so that the emphasis was on educating local physicians rather than on delivering direct care. The meetings at which these changes were discussed got heated and ugly. One somehow devolved into an argument over whether surgeons should be able to bring their families on medical trips (paid for by the surgeon, of course). The new board members seemed really pissed off. During that tiff, one of them said to a longtime volunteer doctor, "You know, the difference between you and me is that you believe the customer is the surgeon, and I believe the customer is the patient." The shocked doctor assured him that wasn't true — that the patient always comes first. The board member's accusation hurt but not as much as the new medical director saying that Interplast volunteers were medical imperialists, pushing aside local physicians in favor of training American residents. That was the direct opposite of what I'd perceived to be happening over three decades.

Deciding whether or not residents and interns should take part in Interplast trips required two contentious board meetings, each more than six hours long. The big objections were that the educating of residents was preventing the education of local surgeons and that the residents and interns were costing Interplast money and weren't contributing directly to the bottom line. Several longtime volunteer supervising surgeons testified to what a tremendously valuable experience Interplast trips were for young surgeons, pediatricians, and anesthesiologists. I reminded the group that since its founding, Interplast had existed not only to provide free reconstructive surgery for needy children and adults in developing nations and to partner with local medical professionals, train them in specialized procedures, and assist them in moving toward medical independence, but also to offer American residents and interns the chance to treat problems they were less likely to encounter at home. That angle had been especially important at Stanford, where our upscale clientele didn't offer enough pathology for plastic and reconstructive surgery residents to learn on. A bonus: Interplast also taught students the value of serving the needy and got them hooked on the psychic income of helping.

I also pointed out to the board that the residents were indeed contributing to the bottom line; it was just that the payoff didn't come until six to ten years down the road when these advanced students became established clinicians, a new generation of Interplast volunteer doctors. Furthermore, I thought that the presence of residents helped, rather than hurt local surgeons: the residents and interns could do clinical intake interviews, data entry, and routine post-op rounds, and they could set up research protocols, meaning the experienced American surgeons were able to concentrate on working with their local counterparts.

The final vote of the board was 15 to 13 in favor of banning residents and interns. I felt bereft. My residents — ultimately, I would mentor fifty-nine of them — were part of my family, as Uncle Hippocrates directed. Most of them participated in Interplast, and those volunteers went on to greater glory. Here are just a few from that roster:

- Robert Pearl, MD, was the CEO of the Permanente Medical Group, heading a team of 9,000 physicians serving four million patients.
- Terry Knapp, MD, cofounded the Collagen Corporation and a series of successful biotech companies.
- Catherine deVries, MD, who traveled with Interplast as a resident in pediatric urology, started the international nonprofit IVUmed, which provides free urologic surgery all over the developing world.
- David Fogarty, MD, DDS, not only traveled all over the globe with Interplast, he started a domestic branch to serve the needy in Appalachia.
- Debra Johnson, MD, is former president of the American Society of Plastic Surgeons.
- William McClure, MD, launched Interplast's Vietnam program. His first Interplast trip, to Honduras, was also his honeymoon; his wife, Chris, is a nurse.
- Joanne Stenger, MD, was the first woman in the innovative six-year joint general surgery/

plastic and reconstructive surgery residency
program that Chase and I started, the first
in the country. (Until then, people interested in
plastic surgery had to do five years of general
surgery training before they could begin
immersing themselves in plastic and reconstructive surgery techniques; now all schools
follow the integrated model.) Joanne had been
a flight attendant and a chemistry teacher
before going to medical school; she traveled
as an Interplast volunteer to Central America,
Mexico, and the South Pacific, and became a
distinguished professor at Stanford.

• Jim Chang, MD, is now the chief of Plastic &
Reconstructive Surgery at Stanford and the
current medical director of ReSurge.

When students applied for a residency in plastic
surgery, they had to produce three stellar letters of rec-
ommendation and write about themselves and their
ambitions. Chase and I thoroughly evaluated their spatial and psychomotor skills (one timed test: placing tiny
beads onto an upturned needle using surgical forceps).
Finally, there came an interview. One of the key questions was "Why did you choose plastic surgery?" One
candidate answered, "I want to have a nice lifestyle." I
told her that she'd given the wrong answer. Immediately
and without loss of aplomb, she asked what the right
answer was and how she could correct herself. I told her
to call Phil at the Latin American Mission Project clinic

in Mexicali and arrange to stay with him for a month to learn Spanish and develop a social conscience. She was down there within a week. Her determination and motivation got her a place in the Stanford program. People like her were being dropped from Interplast by the new board, CEO, and medical director.

The other huge source of tension between longtime volunteers and the new professional staff was the shifting of Interplast's focus from direct service (sending surgeons and other medical professionals overseas to provide reconstructive surgery) to education (investing in training foreign doctors and providing resources and infrastructure so that these local professionals could serve their own population). I felt we were doing that already. Organizational consultants were called in from the Stanford Business School and McKinsey & Company. They believed that focus on training local physicians — through web-based lectures, computer-assisted training, and fellowships that brought them to the U.S. for advanced studies — would give us a competitive advantage over other humanitarian medical groups trying to raise money. Education and empowerment would be our thing. I thought it was already our thing, considering the long list of empowered partner physicians, including Edgar Rodas, an Ecuadoran surgeon who went on to found Cinterandes, a mobile surgery unit that's provided 7,000 operations to rural patients without health services; or Guillermo Peña of Honduras, who has become a world-class craniofacial surgeon. Many spent time at Stanford, such as Cesar

Michaan of Guatemala, who did a yearlong fellowship with Chase.

The newcomers wanted to fix what they saw as a paradox built into the founding mission: we could only ensure the independence of local doctors if we made ourselves obsolete as deliverers of direct care. I, too, hoped that would happen, but I was hurt and bewildered by some statements that the new medical director made, memorialized on video. "You create no infrastructure by going with your good equipment and jumping on a plane and coming home," he said. He didn't seem to know that we left most of our equipment with the host country, and we left a vital store of knowledge, too.

Our rejiggered mission and the new emphasis on web-based curricula went over well with donors, attracting, for example, half a million dollars from Ronald McDonald House. That was great. But I was smarting from the accusations of having failed to create independence and infrastructure in host countries and pained by the absence of residents. I remained vocal in my disagreement. It may be possible that what I regarded as a passionate defense of our original mission was construed by some as cantankerous contrarianism that sabotaged progress. I was ousted from the board of Interplast. Some longtime volunteer doctors and nurses left in solidarity; others didn't.

The ban against residents would ultimately be lifted, and my rift with Interplast/ReSurge International repaired in a way satisfying to all. Back then, though, I felt mad and martyred. I didn't want to fight. And then my energies were claimed by a much bigger battle.

FOURTEEN

THE HISTORY OF MY HEAD

I always seemed to be banging my brainpan. As a toddler, I climbed out of my stroller and toppled noggin-first onto concrete. In grade school, I excelled at a game called Pom-Pom-Pullaway — a sort of hybrid of tag, Red Rover, and human dodgeball — by barreling head-first into my opponents. In junior high and high school, I was the best tackler on the football team. My high school coach urged us all to tackle trees as we walked to and from school.

For me, the art of surgery involves not only technique — doing the operation with elegance, flow, and precision — but also grace and honesty in interacting with patients and colleagues and partnership with a higher power. The basic act is mechanical, but it's informed by the intuitive and the mysterious. I felt the same way about being a good cornerback. The art of tackling, like the art of surgery, only worked if three elements were working in sync — mechanical skill honed by practice, human teamwork, and the element of the mysterious and the intuitive.

The physical pleasure of contact sports became a kind of addiction, and I added boxing to football. The price of this pleasure was a repetitive bouncing around of my brain within the calvarium, the bony skull — and five concussions before college.

Though I mistreated my head, I counted on it (with its partner, my heart) to get me to my goal of healing the world. So, I was deeply alarmed when my head stopped working properly.

Trouble hit at a time when my life was running smoothly. I wasn't happy about the big changes in Interplast, but I figured that an interesting epoch was about to begin. My busy office felt like a vital nerve center. My motto was "Why practice unless you can be the best in the world?" My usual response to "Doctor, we have a problem," was "No problem!" — because I thought I could solve anything. I felt immortal. Years of leading a wildish life seemed to have no detrimental effect on me. I could always drink more, exercise harder, work longer, and stay up later than most. I was intoxicated with the arrogance of success. I felt I was above everybody and that therefore I could abuse my body without consequences.

In late 1999, I underwent a routine physical that included a neurological assessment for stroke. The doctor had me hold both arms out in front of me, parallel to the floor, and keep them exactly side by side for thirty seconds with my eyes closed. When I opened my eyes again, I saw that my left arm had somehow dropped below my right. The doctor declared this to be an infallible sign of stroke. I said, "You must be wrong. Do the test again." He obliged, and this time, I cheated by raising my left arm ever so slightly to compensate for my previous deficiency. I was more concerned about challenging him than about the implications of the test result. I assumed the guy was just plain wrong, and I thought nothing of it.

The summer of 2000 arrived, along with the first prodromal symptoms: a tight feeling in my head; becoming lost while visiting a restaurant men's room in Key West; fainting without obvious cause while I was helping my son Don Jr. build a playhouse for his children in Burlington, Vermont. And then I found myself unable to write the letter g in cursive. It was time to see a neurologist.

The initial diagnosis of my doctor was that I was suffering from depression caused by facing retirement. But just in case, he ordered a brain MRI. It showed more than the usual infarcts — areas of tissue that were dead or dying because an obstruction had deprived them of blood — for a man my age. I consulted another fine neurologist for a second opinion. He knew the radiologist who'd assessed my MRI and felt she'd "overread" the scan.

But day by day I became worse and worse. I spent hours lying on the couch in front of the fireplace in a sort of stupor. On the advice of my physicians, Judy and my daughter Julie brought me to the University of California, San Francisco (UCSF) Medical Center. The neurologist who saw me believed that I had something more serious than a stroke and that a complete workup was necessary to arrive at a precise diagnosis. But there was no room in the hospital for immediate admission. The neurologist told my wife and daughter that if there was real trouble while I was waiting to be admitted, they should bring me directly to the emergency room.

On Christmas Eve in 2000, Judy and Julie did just that, driving thirty miles north in a mighty rainstorm, with me lying in the back seat. We were met by the chief resident in neurology and the doctor I'd seen earlier. That first night in the hospital, I dreamed there was a huge party for me on New Year's Eve, my birthday, with drinking and dancing and happy hugging. When I awoke, I thought I was in a hotel in Santa Cruz because I could hear the surf, which turned out to be the sound of the air conditioning at UCSF.

I underwent a battery of tests, and doctors diagnosed prion disease, a.k.a. mad cow, universally fatal. "We'll discharge you tomorrow for home care and rest," I was told. "Later we'll arrange for your transfer to a hospice, where they'll relieve your pain with morphine sulfate. The short remainder of your life on earth will be peaceful."

Before I left, the doctors wanted to document my case for research purposes. They asked for permission to do a brain biopsy — to take a sample of my brain tissue. Dr. Michael McDermott appeared at my bedside. He was terrifically smart, technically proficient, well dressed, and confident, with a nice neat mustache. I asked him, "How high up in the faculty are you?" He snorted. "High enough for you." I asked how many of these biopsies he had performed. "Ten thousand," he said. We were both familiar with the old one-upmanship routine. I felt I was in good hands.

I awoke and felt staples in my scalp. Dr. McDermott reported that my brain looked like a toad, with small orange-colored bumps all over it. Frozen-section pathology showed malignancy, probably lymphoma, but the exact type would require more investigation. No sooner had he delivered the alarming news than the oncology team descended upon me for further diagnostic tests. The verdict: I had a case of intravascular large B-cell lymphoma, an aggressive cancer of the blood that affects B-lymphocytes, a type of white blood cell that serves the immune system by producing antibodies. The cancer wasn't in the brain tissue itself but inside multiple small blood vessels. Small tumors had begun to shut off the blood supply in the same way a stroke might; this blockage created the symptoms and scan results that caused confusion before I was correctly diagnosed.

The lead oncologist told me, "This is a rare cancer. There are only two hundred cases in the literature, with twenty still alive. We've had three at this hospital, with one still alive." No standard protocol existed, so the oncology team reviewed all the literature and proposed an autologous stem cell transplant — harvesting of my own stem cells from the bone marrow — and a chemotherapy regimen that included a new "smart bomb" drug designed to attack my particular breed of lymphoma.

For some reason, I felt neither terror nor panic at the

diagnosis or the proposed treatment, which offered only a 15 percent chance of survival, if I weathered the complications. When I realized that the odds were that I was scheduled to lose my physical life, I thought, *This won't hurt. It will be pleasant. It's another adventure, like a ride at Great America that goes into a pitch-black tunnel and before releasing you presents opportunities to build character, to improve yourself. When I come out the other side, it will all be pastel, no anxiety, and all the nice people will rendezvous.* I planned to buy a first-class Bordeaux as soon as possible. I had in my mind a nice rock in the sun to sit on.

For a second opinion, I invited advice from the world's foremost expert on lymphoma, Professor Saul Rosenberg at Stanford. Judy and Julie accompanied me. Saul said that he'd gone over my case with his clinic staff. "You have a mortality expectation of 70 percent with chemotherapy and a stem cell transplant," he said. "You'll have some brain damage, but your brain can stand it. You'll probably get mucositis, where you can't swallow, and your entire GI tract mucosa may slough out." He cited other possible complications from treatment, pulmonary and infectious, all associated with the probability that I would die.

As we parted, he said gently and jokingly, "You know, when you took off that basal cell cancer from my nose, you left too much nose." We all laughed. He embraced me, and I thought that he was crying as he left the room. He seemed to be saying, "This is it." Part of me was ready to agree and say, "Okay, my life is finished. I'm at the jumping-off place." But a stronger, more standard reaction kicked in: whenever there's a situation in which I should say no because too much trouble lies ahead, I feel a powerful need to say yes. I always figure I'll deal later with any problems or roadblocks. I said yes to treatment. I had a desire for the experience.

My life was saved by hotshot oncologists who gave me six courses of smart bomb chemotherapy and an autologous stem cell transplant — the harvesting, freezing, and reintroduction of my own stem cells from the bone marrow where they're manufactured. These undifferentiated cells, the body's repair kit, could later be turned into healthy lymphocytes, replacing the cancerous ones killed by chemo.

First came a round of heavy-duty chemotherapy to wipe out all the white blood cells produced by my bone marrow in order to stop the aberrant and uncontrolled growth of B-lymphocytes. Good, helpful cells were killed along with the villains — collateral damage. My white blood cell count fell to zero, leaving my body defenseless against infection for a few days. Then I was given a white-blood-cell stimulating hormone, and my white-cell count jumped to normal and beyond. Doctors placed a catheter in my jugular vein to collect blood and centrifuged it to separate out the stem cells. I was proud that I gave them more than the expected twenty-four million. These cells were then stored at -300°F for later reintroduction. After harvest came five more rounds of scorched-earth chemo. All of my body's lymphocytes were wiped out. I was nearly wiped out, as well. Several days later, the first five million stem cells were returned to my body by a cheerful nurse bearing a 6occ syringe. She found one of the last veins left from chemo and injected the stem cells, which in effect began saving my life within five minutes. The illness well and truly scrambled my head. I have little memory of the period from Thanksgiving of 2000 to the second week of January 2001, although occasional cameo experiences flash through. Here are some of the things I *don't* remember but have been told — stories about my behavior when I was still under the influence of various pathogens and chemicals. Awakening from the brain biopsy, I was apprehended in the process of pulling out all the tubes from my veins and bladder. I attempted to jump off the back of the bed, with my son Don holding me and Judy shouting "Nooo, Don! Nooo, Don!" Apparently, I replied, "I don't want to hear 'Nooo, Don!' ever again for the rest of my life, goddammit!"

My wonderfully patient nurses reported that when I was trying to use the urine bottle in bed, I failed because I insisted on placing the device on my abdomen rather than between the legs. Then I looked around and found one of my long cotton socks and attempted to use that, but it leaked. In order to solve my problem, I staggered to the nurses' station and asked for a rubber glove. Back in bed, I easily filled it with urine and tied it off. Having finally accomplished this monumental task, I then took the fat little five-legged creature to the nurses' station and plopped it on the counter. They drew a smiley face on it with a magic marker.

Here's one thing I do remember. I was lying in my

hospital bed recovering from the third course of scorched-earth chemo, dreaming deeply. I awoke at dawn with the dream still in my mind, and it remains vivid to this day.

I'm a young faculty member at Stanford, on the hand-surgery service of Dr. Chase, running the residency training program. He's asked me to do a "special case" — a young male business executive with a trigger finger. (That's tenosynovitis, or inflammation of the tendon. The tendon runs through a pulley system, which becomes too tight when the sheath and tendon are inflamed, contracting the finger into a claw.)

Dr. Chase introduces me to the patient — a tall, husky man in a light blue silk suit. Then Chase asks privately that I train eight residents on this case — four I know, and four new ones. The new residents are black wolves. But they're nice wolves, very intelligent, very handsome, and already partially trained. The four human residents and I have never met these wolf-doctors before. I feel pressure, because of the precision necessary for any hand surgery, the attention required for the training of residents, and the anxiety associated with training four wolves to do surgery.

The human residents and I had fetched the patient in my old green pickup truck, which was loaded as usual with mushroom compost. The humans are well prepared; they've studied up on trigger finger surgery, done the preoperative workup to evaluate the possible causes of the condition, and explored the possible presence of other clinical conditions that may affect the patient outcome. They've also administered informed consent, evaluated the lab work, given antibiotics, and prepared the operating room to per-fection. We're ready for any eventuality.

In the operating room, that sacred place, the black wolves are well behaved and seem somewhat famil-iar with standard operating procedure and OR politics. But I worry about their knowledge of sterile technique, and I'm anxious about whether or not I can teach them surgery with their lack of prehensile abilities. Walking around the perimeter of the room, I bump into one par-ticularly smart, accommodating black wolf who weighs over 200 pounds. His full heft hits my midsection, and the collision doesn't feel good.

At that instant, I awoke to the real world and began to wonder about the meaning of the dream and why I hadn't been allowed to finish it. I can recall thinking that it was ridiculous to relate the dream to any previous episode in my life — my adolescent interest in wolves, say, or my pride in my residents, or my sorrow at having them excluded from Interplast trips. I also felt that the dream couldn't have any psychiatric interpretation. Those thoughts seem particularly misguided, in retrospect.

Was the dream a reminder of the promise to serve the world that I made as a terrified fourteen-year-old certain he was going to be eaten by wolves? Was it a recap of my medical career, or an affirmation of my ability to handle any situation? Did it reflect anxiety about the unknown and unforeseen, or acceptance that such things were a part of life that I could handle? Was it the fulfillment of a wish to tame the untamable? Was it about interdepend-ence, commonality of purpose, trusting the team? About the ways that being dangerously ill meant colliding with my animal nature? I think of wolves as characterized by confidence, aggression, competitiveness, mental strength, strength of spirit, cleverness, teamwork ability, valor, courage, survivability — precisely the characteristics that I looked for in my residents. Therefore, these select members of two different species were easily able to work together and they indeed were even useful to each other's purpose. In any case, it was a good dream, and I had the strength of wolves — I got better.

It can take two to three weeks after an autologous transplant for the stem cells to find their old home in the marrow and start a factory to produce healthy blood cells. Recovery takes two to four months; returning to a normal activity level takes even longer. Fifty days after chemotherapy began, I experienced the complication of reactive chemical pneumonitis, which required high dose of prednisone once a day for ten days. But I was getting better and better.

What had caused the cancer? Was it the head trauma from football and boxing? Huge doses of UV radiation during high school and college summers working construction without wearing a hat or shirt? The fact that I didn't eat my veggies for the first thirty-five years of my life? The herbicide I sprayed regularly on our kiwifruit orchard? Some genetic cellular weakness?

And what if boxing and football had toughened me up, rather than wrecked my head? What if my survival was assisted by the fact that I listened to Burl Ives on my Sony Walkman day and night? Did I make it through because once I was diagnosed, I decided never to worry about the prognosis but rather to be accepting, be courageous, and just deal with it?

For me, the question remained: if only very few have survived this condition, why did I live? I asked four experienced oncologists, and all of them gave essentially the same answers: I experienced a good outcome because I had access to cutting-edge medical treatments; intense, loving support from family (Judy shaved her head in solidarity) and friends (some of whom sneaked a porterhouse steak and a briefcase full of beer into my hospital room); faith in prayer (and not just those of family and friends — one online pastor had 2,000 parishioners pray for my benefit); a new, good diet; and an ornery personality. I would add, in fairness to all much-loved, stubborn, abstemious people of faith who died from this disease despite top-notch treatment, the luck of the draw.

But I also felt, very strongly, that I lived because I had more work to do.

FIFTEEN

DOCTORGENARIAN

The first work of my second life was recovery. Home from the hospital, I had nursing care and then a baby-sitter — an aide who helped me go to the bathroom or get a drink of water. I also had him catalog my hundreds of books. I think I was launching, in an inchoate way, a kind of life inventory. When I could manage more movement, a personal trainer did exercises with me. And as my physical health improved, I had the urge to do manual labor, something I'd loved as a teenager. I started helping a contractor build a guest house on our property. If ever again we had doctors from Chile, Vietnam, and Turkey staying with us at the same time, we'd have plenty of room for them. That guest house turned out to be a gorgeous thing — and ridiculously expensive. It helped heal me and broke the family bank.

Recovery from brain cancer meant a renewed appreciation for life's blessings, and the need to cope with its blows. The greatest of those: I could no longer perform surgery. I had to find new ways to serve, new sources of meaning. I began teaching courses at Stanford Medical School in international humanitarian medicine, which was deeply rewarding because of the people I met and the multiplier effect as class after class of medical students enthusiastically took part in various programs abroad, including, of course, Interplast/ReSurge. I also did consulting for gender dysphoria practices. A few years after my illness, I was invited to visit a large conference on gender confirmation surgery in San Francisco, run by the transgender community. I worried that I would be considered an outsider there, but the opposite was the case. The warmth and appreciation expressed by members of the community made my spirits soar.

In 2017, my enthusiastic embrace of risk in the name of humane medical innovation was the subject of an episode of the NPR podcast *Hidden Brain*. The host, journalist Shankar Vedantam, noted that the Greek poet Archilochus wrote, "The fox knows many things, but the hedgehog knows one big thing." Psychologists, he said, use this epigram to define two cognitive styles: foxes are comfortable with nuance and can live with contradictions; they use different strategies for different situations. Hedgehogs, on the other hand, focus on the big picture, the big idea. They're decisive, they're leaders, and, he said, they solve every problem with one basic organizing principle. I was happy to be presented as the exemplary hedgehog, though I'd say that *my* basic life principle — do a big thing and help a lot of people — has undergone an alteration since my recovery from lymphoma, a C-change, as it were.

I still think taking risks in order to serve others is a terrific idea; one of the key sub-principles in my stealth manifesto remains "do the impossible." I'll never let go of the motto "think outside the box" (although I long ago accepted the corollary added by my wise, beautiful, unflappable wife: ". . . but always keep one foot inside the box for balance and stability"). Here's what's changed: I no longer need to be the absolute best at something — surgery, or humanitarian service, or kayaking, or tackling trees. Competitiveness and one-upmanship have lost their luster. Through the lens of cancer, I see clearly that the most important things in life are the relationships we have with family and friends. And the world is full of my friends — who are really my family. Your blood is my blood; your cells are my cells — that's how I think now. Life is more enjoyable than before.

My statistically miraculous remission has lasted nearly two decades, though not without some scars. The damage caused by the cancer and the chemo intermittently affects my decision-making, mood, and memory. There's a passage in *Gratitude*, the last book written by the extraordinary neurologist Oliver Sacks and published posthumously, that moves me: ". . . the events of the world . . . are experienced and constructed in a highly subjective way. . . . Our only truth is narrative truth, the stories we tell each other and ourselves — the stories we continually recategorize and refine." Writing this memoir — in fact, living my second life — has been an exercise in recategorization and refinement by means of my own ruminations, with the assistance of archival evidence and the collective memories of family, friends, and colleagues, including the residents I've mentored. All of these people continually enrich my treasury of stories.

I believe our spirits live forever even after our bodies are no more. I believe that real prayer is always answered, although the answer doesn't always correspond to the request and may not be understandable until much later. Or ever. People get frustrated with having to die, but what the hell? It's another adventure. (One that I don't feel compelled to embark upon right this minute, I hasten to say. I think of St. Augustine: "Give me chastity and continence, but not just yet.")

I'm in my eighties now and thinking about signs, portents, and legacy. Among the good signs and portents: the *Time* magazine cover in June 2014 featuring the beautiful trans actress and activist Laverne Cox and the words *The Transgender Tipping Point: America's Next Civil Rights Frontier.* I know that the 1.5 million Americans who identify as transgender still have a tough row to hoe, but California and ten other states now provide insurance for gender confirmation surgery, and the year 2017 brought some milestones: in North Carolina, the ridiculous "bathroom bill" was repealed. In California, new legislation requires insurance companies to cover gender confirmation surgery. And President Trump's out-of-the-blue, ill-informed, misguided, and short-sighted presidential order banning transgender people from the military was ignored by the Pentagon.

Furthermore, though no definitive answers are in yet, marvelous new research points to a biological cause for gender dysphoria. For example, scientists know that there are some structural differences between the brains of females and males. Researchers in Spain have used MRI to show that transgender people have brains more similar to their experienced gender than to their gender at birth. Similarly, neuroscientists in the Netherlands, aware that a certain steroid causes a different response in the hypo-thalamus of males and females, found that adolescent girls and boys with gender dysphoria responded physically to the steroid in ways expected of their experienced gender rather than their birth gender.

As for legacy, the most precious to me is my chil-dren. I once told an interviewer that I found my family life paradoxically perfect and awful. Perfect, because we all enjoyed one another so much, and awful because I was gone a lot. At a roast my friends and colleagues gave me, my son Don jokingly showed what he said was his favorite photo of me from his childhood. It was the rear end of my Cadillac going out the driveway. But the kids seem to have matured unscathed, and we had plenty of family fun. All of them went on Interplast trips through-out Central and South America, starting when they were ten or so. I put them to work filing or keeping supplies stocked. And now it can be told: since I wasn't much of a fellow for rules, I allowed them to observe in the OR, gowned and masked. I wanted to make sure they all caught the spirit of Interplast, and they did, sticking with it as adults. Ray went on several Interplast trips as official photographer, and he also documented surgery for the Gender Dysphoria Program. He now lives on the Big Island of Hawaii, where he grows avocados, guava, and cocoa. Donald Jr. is a plastic and reconstructive surgeon who exceeds me in every way. He's been a volunteer on many international medical missions. Mary became a nurse and volunteered with Interplast in Vietnam and Peru; she's now a hospice nurse. Julie, who manages an interior design store, and Louise, a graphic designer, have also volunteered on international medical trips.

I had two compulsions in my professional life — to even out the inequities in medical services between the developed and developing world and to use surgery to relieve the suffering caused by gender dysphoria. Those worked out pretty well, legacy-wise.

Since its inception fifty years ago, Interplast/ReSurge's multidisciplinary teams of physicians and those of its sister organizations have performed 200,000 life-changing surgeries in fifteen countries, establishing thousands of long-term relationships with physicians all over the world. I personally participated in 1,500 cleft lip and palate surgeries during 159 Interplast trips on five continents. The original spirit of Interplast/ReSurge has given rise to fifty-eight independent university- or foundation-based humanitarian surgical organizations including Interplast

Germany, Interplast Turkey, Interplast Holland, Interplast Italy, Interplast Australia, Interplast West Virginia, One Heart World-Wide, IVUmed, and more. They all carry out my vision of healing the world through plastic surgery. The World Health Organization (WHO) has declared that access to medical care is a human right and that the unavailability of healthcare is a root cause of extreme poverty. WHO doesn't explicitly mention surgery, but according to its own figures, two billion people lack access to basic surgical care; more people die from unmet surgical need than from AIDS and malaria and other ailments combined. I intend to go out hollering that access to surgery is a human right.

As for the nearly 1,500 gender affirmation surgeries I performed and the care that followed, the lasting joy of that legacy is encapsulated in a message I recently received on my web page:

> Dr. Laub, you made my life worth living.
> (Stanford, 1980s.)

> Signed,
> An Early One

ACKNOWLEDGMENTS

My grateful thanks to the heart and soul of Interplast, social workers Amy Laden and Judy Van Maasdam, and to the spirit of the Laub clan: Judy McCotter Laub, R1 Ray H. Laub, D2 Donald Laub II, R2 Ray T. Laub, Julieann Laub, Mary Holmes Laub, and Louise Carolita Laub. The spirit of the clan shines brightly from Judith Stone, editor-in-chief; Bill McClure, Dick Jobe, Francis Small JD, Ernie Kaplan, and John and Bianca Zimmermann. These are persons with whom I have formed a deep relationship by virtue of our work together.

Others include . . .

. . . humanitarian surgeons who significantly contributed to the world of Interplasts: Jaroy Weber Jr., David G. Dibbell, Lars M. Vistnes, Dave Fogarty, Terry Knapp,

Mark Gorney, Richard J. Siegel, Vincent R. Hentz, Steve Schendel, Richard Ott, Roberto Palma, Bill Magee, Angelo Capozzi, Evaleen Jones, Larry Nichter, Gottfried Lemperle, Minay Kurtai, Shankar Rai, Sunil Richardson, Namik Baran, Debra Johnson, Paul Daines, Jon Daines, Jorge Palacios, Glenn Geelhoed, Catherine DeVries.

. . . my inner circle of international humanitarian surgeons each of whom has started their own foundations which have each performed more than 5,000 operations: Edgar Rodas, Javier Beut, Gottfried Lemperle, Andre Borsche, Paolo Morselli, Jaime Caloca, Qadir Ghulam Fayyaz, Shankar Rai, Sunil Richardson, Namik Baran, Oscar Asensio, Eid Mustafa.

. . . experienced anesthesiologists and nurses: David Vernon Thomas, Murray Walker, Loren Eltherington, "Lord" Gordon Taylor.

. . . huge professional patrons each with a specific discipline: Phillip Collins, Bill Lazier, Andrea Jobe, Sue Ewens, Keith Walter, Margrit Elliot, Gene Gaynor, Katherine Wright, Linda Farrell, Richard Frye, Jim Southern, George Chippendale, Chuck Swanson.

In addition, I'd like to acknowledge the following people for their indispensible support: David Werner, Ed Walsh, SJ Vettam, Rocio Molina, Doreen Molina, the team at ECW — Jack David, Jen Hale, and Jen Albert — and my agent, Sheree Bykofsky.

Finally, I want to pay homage to those on whose principles I base my work:

For the good of the whole rather than the individual
— CONFUCIUS

Improve yourself with skill and knowledge
for the benefit of the other person
— HIPPOCRATES

Love your neighbor as yourself
— SECOND COMMANDMENT OF JESUS CHRIST

Respect for all living things
— DR. & REV ALBERT SCHWEITZER

In medicine, investigate both the social and
the physical disabilities
— DR. PAUL BRAND

Inviting medical personnel from hostile countries to
train together is the first step toward peace in the world
— DR. CHARLES HORTON

Consider the patient as the boss in your
decision-making
— DR. ROBERT CHASE

Provide surgery to those who don't have access to it
— DR. TOM DOOLEY

Medical care is a universal human right
— DR. JAMES TURPIN

Do the right thing
— JUDY LAUB

ABOUT THE AUTHOR

Donald R. Laub Sr., MD, is a retired plastic and reconstructive surgeon who was Chief of Plastic Surgery at Stanford University School of Medicine from 1968 to 1980 before entering private practice.

He is the founder of Interplast (now called ReSurge International), the first nonprofit medical charity to send multidisciplinary surgical teams to perform transformative plastic and reconstructive surgery free of charge in the developing world.

Laub is also a pioneer in gender affirmation surgery. From 1981 to 1983, Laub was president of the organization now known as the World Professional Association for Transgender Health and participated in drafting the international *Standards of Care for the Health of*

Transsexual, Transgender, and Gender Nonconforming People.

In 2013, Laub was given the American College of Surgeons' Surgical Humanitarian Award, "in recognition of those surgeons who have dedicated a substantial portion of their career to ensuring the provision of surgical care to underserved populations without expectation of commensurate reimbursement." And in 2017, he was presented with the prestigious President's Honorary Citation, bestowed by the American Society of Plastic Surgeons. Laub is the coauthor of *The Alternate-Day Diet* (TarcherPerigee, 2013). He lives in California near Stanford University with his wife, Judy.

At ECW Press, we want you to enjoy this book in whatever format you like, whenever you like. Leave your print book at home and take the eBook to go! Purchase the print edition and receive the eBook free. Just send an email to ebook@ecwpress.com and include:

- the book title
- the name of the store where you purchased it
- your receipt number
- your preference of file type: PDF or ePub?

A real person will respond to your email with your eBook attached. And thanks for supporting an independently owned Canadian publisher with your purchase!